ESSENTIALS *of* PATHOPHYSIOLOGY *for* PHARMACY

CRC PRESS PHARMACY EDUCATION SERIES

Pharmaceutical Care: Insights from Community Pharmacists
William N. Tindall and Marsha K. Millonig

Essentials of Law and Ethics for Pharmacy Technicians
Kenneth M. Strandberg

Essentials of Pharmacy Law
Douglas J. Pisano

Essentials of Pathophysiology for Pharmacy
Martin M. Zdanowicz

Pharmac y: What It Is and How It Works
William N. Kelly

Pharmacokinetic Principles of Dosing Adjustments: Understanding the Basics
Ronald Schoenwald

Strauss's Federal Drug Laws and Examination Review, Fifth Edition
Steven Strauss

Pharmaceutical and Clinical Calculations, Second Edition
Mansoor Khan and Indra Reddy

Inside Pharmacy: Anatomy of a Profession
Ray Gosselin, Jack Robbins, and Joseph Cupolo

Understanding Medical Terms: A Guide for Pharmacy Practice, Second Edition
Mary Stanaszek, Walter Stanaszek, and Robert Holt

Pharmacokinetic Analysis: A Practical Approach
Peter Lee and Gordon Amidon

Guidebook for Patient Counseling
Harvey Rappaport, Tracey Hunter, Joseph Roy, and Kelly Straker

ESSENTIALS *of* PATHOPHYSIOLOGY *for* PHARMACY

MARTIN M. ZDANOWICZ

CRC PRESS

Boca Raton London New York Washington, D.C.

Library of Congress Cataloging-in-Publication Data

Zdanowicz, Martin M.
Essentials of pathophysiology for pharmacy / by Martin M. Zdanowicz
p. ; cm.-- (CRC Press pharmacy education series)
Includes bibliographical references and index.
ISBN 1-58716-036-6 (alk. paper)
1. Physiology, Pathological. I. Title. II. Series.
[DNLM: 1. Pathology--methods. 2. Physiology--methods. 3. Drug Therapy--methods.
QZ 140 Z396e 2002]
RB113 .Z337 2002
616.07--dc21 2002067061

Direct all inquiries to CRC Press LLC, 2000 N.W. Corporate Blvd., Boca Raton, Florida 33431.

Visit the CRC Press Web site at www.crcpress.com

International Standard Book Number 1-58716-036-6
Library of Congress Card Number 2002067061
Printed in the United States of America 1 2 3 4 5 6 7 8 9 0
Printed on acid-free paper

Dedication

This book is lovingly dedicated to my wife Christine, my son Alex, and my daughter Olivia, who are my constant joy and inspiration. I would also like to dedicate this book to the students for constantly bringing out the best in me. I only hope that I am able to bring out the best in them…

You cannot depend on your eyes when your imagination is out of focus.

— Mark Twain

Preface

This book was written as a clear, concise learning instrument for students in pharmacy or sciences. Many of the large pathophysiology textbooks used today are very detailed works that often include chapters on normal physiology and function, topics that are redundant for pharmacy or health science students who will take separate courses in human physiology as part of their curriculum.

The book begins with an overview of tissue injury and mechanisms of tissue repair to provide students with a foundation of key concepts in injury and repair that appear throughout subsequent chapters. A detailed discussion of the immune system is also included early on because this system plays a key role in a number of important disease processes. The discussion of the immune system is followed by an up-to-date discussion of HIV that includes important information regarding HIV mutation and drug resistance.

The book continues with a detailed presentation of diseases affecting the main organ systems including cardiovascular, respiratory, renal, gastrointestinal, hepatic and endocrine disorders. The book concludes with a comprehensive look at diabetes mellitus.

The presentation of material within the chapters is designed to maximize clarity and facilitate conveyance of key points to the students. Subsections, bulleted lists, tables and definitions of key terms are included in each chapter along with study objectives that are designed to focus students on important concepts within each chapter. Each chapter includes a rationale for drug therapy section that allows students to correlate information they have learned on selected diseases to the clinical application of drugs. The author's experience in teaching both pathophysiology and pharmacology has made it clear that the time to introduce pharmacy and health science students to therapeutics is with the study of pathophysiology, where the mechanism and effects of disease are explored in detail. The presentation of drug therapy in this book is general and in most cases does not focus on the uses of specific drugs within a class but rather on a class of drugs as a whole. The goal of the drug therapy section is to expose students to various drug classes with emphasis on how these drug classes are used to treat a specific disease state. Major side effects of these drug classes are also included. However, specific drug nomenclature and dosing are not included, nor are detailed mechanisms of drug action because these topics will be covered in detail in subsequent pharmacology and therapeutics classes.

Although this book was designed as a stand-alone text for a pathophysiology course in a pharmacy or health sciences program, it may also be useful as a clear and concise supplement to some of the larger, more comprehensive textbooks that are currently available. This book may also serve as an excellent review of pathophysiology for students preparing for standardized exams or for anyone who needs to update his or her knowledge in this area.

Martin M. Zdanowicz

Contents

Chapter 3 Disorders of hemostasis and coagulation

Chapter 4 Alterations in hematologic function and oxygen transport

Chapter 5 Immune response and inflammation

chapter one

Cellular injury

Study objectives

- Compare and contrast the various forms of cellular adaptation. What is the purpose of these adaptive changes?
- Discuss the two underlying mechanisms by which cellular injury can occur.
- List the various classifications of cellular injury that can occur and give examples of each.
- Describe the major manifestations that present when cells are injured. Why does each of these manifestations occur?
- Define apoptosis and necrotic cell death. How do they differ?
- List the specific types of cellular necrosis that may occur along with their distinct characteristics.
- Define gangrene and gas gangrene.
- Discuss the two mechanisms by which tissue repair occurs. Give examples of specific cell types that will utilize each repair mechanism.
- List the steps involved in wound repair along with the key features of each step.
- List various factors that can impair wound healing.
- What is a keloid scar? Why does it occur?

Introduction

The environment around cells is dynamic and constantly changing. In this fluid environment, cells are exposed to numerous stimuli, some of which may be injurious. To survive, cells must have the ability to adapt to variable conditions. This process of adaptation can involve changes in cellular size, number or type.

Cellular adaptation (see Figure 1.1)

1. Atrophy
   - Decrease in size of a cell or tissue.
   - Decreased size results in decreased oxygen consumption and metabolic needs of the cells and may increase the overall efficiency of cell function.
   - Atrophy is generally a reversible process, except for atrophy caused by loss of nervous innervation to a tissue.
   - Causes of atrophy include prolonged bed rest, disuse of limbs or tissue, poor tissue nutrition and ischemia.
2. Hypertrophy
   - Increase in cell size and tissue mass.
   - Occurs when a cell or tissue is exposed to an increased workload.
   - Occurs in tissues that cannot increase cell number as an adaptive response.
   - Hypertrophy may be a normal physiologic response, such as the increase in muscle mass that is seen with exercise, or it may

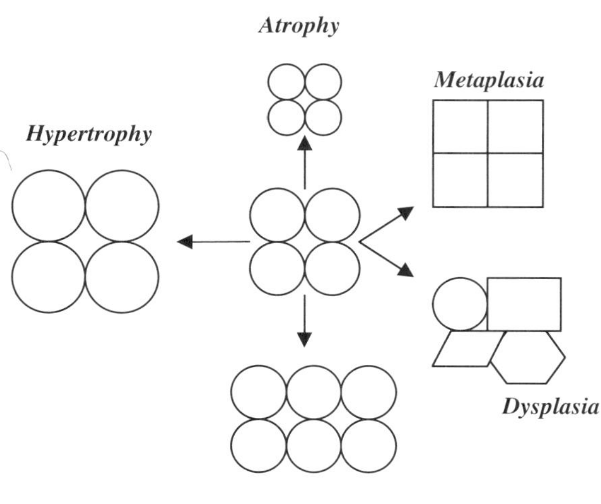

Figure 1.1 Adaptive changes in cells.

be pathologic as in the case of the cardiac hypertrophy that is seen with prolonged hypertension. Hypertrophy may also be a compensatory process. When one kidney is removed, for example, the remaining kidney hypertrophies to increase its functional capacity.

3. Hyperplasia
   - Increase in the number of cells in an organ or tissue.
   - Can only occur in cells capable of mitosis (therefore, not muscle or nerve cells).
   - Hyperplasia may be a normal process, as in the breast and uterine hyperplasia that occurs during pregnancy, or pathologic such as the gingival hyperplasia (overgrowth of gum tissues) that may be seen in certain patients receiving the drug phenytoin.[1] As with hypertrophy, hyperplasia may also be a compensatory mechanism. For example, when a portion of the liver is surgically removed, the remaining hepatocytes (liver cells) increase in number to preserve the functional capacity of the liver.
4. Metaplasia
   - The conversion of one cell type to another cell type that might have a better chance of survival under certain circumstances.
   - Metaplasia usually occurs in response to chronic irritation or inflammation.
   - An example of metaplasia occurs in the respiratory passages of chronic cigarette smokers. Following years of exposure to irritating cigarette smoke, the ciliated columnar epithelium lining the respiratory passages gradually converts to stratified squamous epithelium. Although the stratified squamous cells may be better able to survive the constant irritation of cigarette smoke, they lack the cilia of the columnar epithelial cells that are necessary for clearing particulates from the surfaces of the respiratory passages.
5. Dysplasia
   - A derangement of cell growth that leads to tissues with cells of varying size, shape and appearance.
   - Generally occurs in response to chronic irritation and inflammation.
   - Dysplasia may be a strong precursor to cancer in certain instances such as in the cervix or respiratory tract.

Cellular injury

Cellular injury can occur in a number of different ways. The extent of injury that cells experience is often related to the intensity and duration of exposure to the injurious event or substance. Cellular injury may be a reversible process, in which case the cells can recover their normal function, or it may be irreversible and lead to cell death. Although the causes of cellular injury are many (see Table 1.1), the underlying mechanisms of cellular injury usually fall into one of two categories: *free radical injury* or *hypoxic injury.*

Table 1.1 Classification of Cellular Injury

Physical injury
Mechanical trauma
Temperature extremes (burn injury, frostbite)
Electrical current
Chemical injury
Chemicals, toxins, heavy metals, solvents, smoke, pollutants, drugs, gases
Radiation injury
Ionizing radiation — gamma rays, X rays
Non-ionizing radiation — microwaves, infrared, laser
Biologic agents
Bacteria, viruses, parasites
Nutritional injury
Malnutrition
Obesity

Free radical injury

- Free radicals are highly reactive chemical species that have one or more unpaired electrons in their outer shell.
- Examples of free radicals include *superoxide* (O_2^-), *hydroxyl radicals* (OH^-) and *hydrogen peroxide* (H_2O_2).
- Free radicals are generated as by-products of normal cell metabolism and are inactivated by free radical–scavenging enzymes within the body such as *catalase* and *glutathione peroxidase*. When excess free radicals are formed from exogenous sources or the free radical protective mechanisms fail, injury to cells can occur.
- Free radicals are highly reactive and can injure cells through:
  1. Peroxidation of membrane lipids
  2. Damage of cellular proteins
  3. Mutation of cellular DNA
- Exogenous sources of free radicals include tobacco smoke, organic solvents, pollutants, radiation and pesticides.
- Free radical injury has been implicated as playing a key role in the normal aging process as well as in a number of disease states such as diabetes mellitus, cancer, atheroscelrosis, Alzheimer's disease and rheumatoid arthritis.[2,3]

Hypoxic cell injury

- Hypoxia is a lack of oxygen in cells and tissues that generally results from ischemia.
- During periods of hypoxia, aerobic metabolism of the cells begins to fail. This loss of aerobic metabolism leads to dramatic decreases in energy production (ATP) within the cells. Hypoxic cells begin to swell

as energy-driven processes (such as ATP-driven ion pumps) begin to fail. The pH of the extracellular environment begins to decrease as waste products (such as lactic acid, a product of anaerobic metabolism) begin to accumulate. The cellular injury process may be reversible, if oxygen is quickly restored, or irreversible and lead to cell death. Certain tissues such as the brain are particularly sensitive to hypoxic injury. Death of brain tissues can occur only 4 to 6 minutes after hypoxia begins.

- The loss of ionic balance in hypoxic cells can also lead to the accumulation of intracellular calcium, which is normally closely regulated within cells. There are a number of *calcium-dependent protease* enzymes present within cells that become activated in the presence of excess calcium and begin to digest important cellular constituents.

Manifestations of cellular injury

1. Cellular swelling
   - Caused by an accumulation of water due to the failure of energy-driven ion pumps. Breakdown of cell membrane integrity and accumulation of cellular electrolytes may also occur.
   - Cellular swelling is considered to be a reversible change.
2. Cellular accumulations
   - In addition to water, injured cells can accumulate a number of different substances as metabolism and transport processes begin to fail.
   - Substances that can be accumulated in injured cells may include fats, proteins, glycogen, calcium, uric acid and certain pigments such as melanin.
   - These accumulations are generally reversible but can indicate a greater degree of cellular injury. Accumulation of these substances can be so marked that enlargement of a tissue or organ may occur (for example, fatty accumulation in an injured liver).

Cell death

Cell death falls into two main categories: *apoptosis* and *necrotic cell death*.

Apoptosis

- A controlled, "preprogrammed" cell death that occurs with aging and normal wear and tear of the cell.
- Apoptosis may be a mechanism to eliminate worn-out or genetically damaged cells. Certain viral infections (the Epstein–Barr virus, for example) may activate apoptosis within an infected cell, thus killing both the host cell and infecting virus.

- Apoptosis may involve the activation of certain "suicide genes," which in response to certain chemical signals activate and lead to cell lysis and destruction.
- It has been theorized that cancer may arise as a failure of normal apoptosis in damaged or mutated cells.

Necrotic cell death

- Involves the unregulated, enzymatic digestion ("autolysis") of a cell and its components.
- Occurs as a result of irreversible cellular injury.
- Different types of tissues tend to undergo different types of necrosis. Three main types of necrosis have been identified (see Table 1.2).

Gangrene is the clinical term used when a large area of tissue undergoes necrosis. Gangrene may be classified as *dry gangrene* or *wet gangrene*. With dry gangrene, the skin surrounding the affected area shrinks, wrinkles and turns black. In contrast, wet gangrene presents with an area that is cold, wet from tissue exudates and swollen. A gas gangrene may also occur if the area of necrosis becomes infected with bacteria that produce gases as a by-product.

Tissue repair

Injured or damaged tissues can be repaired in one of two ways, by *regeneration* or *connective tissue replacement*. The mechanism used for repair will depend upon the type of cells that were injured. Certain cells in the body are fully or partially capable of regenerating after an injury, whereas other cell types are not and can only be replaced with connective (scar) tissue.

Table 1.2 Types of Cellular Necrosis

Liquefaction necrosis
Digestive enzymes released by necrotic cells soften and liquefy dead tissue.
Occurs in tissues, such as the brain, that are rich in hydrolytic enzymes.
Caseous necrosis
Dead tissue takes on a crumbly, "cheeselike" appearance. Dead cells disintegrate but their debris is not fully digested by hydrolytic enzymes.
Occurs in conditions like tuberculosis where there is prolonged inflammation and immune activity.
Coagulative necrosis
Dead tissues appear firm, gray and slightly swollen.
Often occurs when cell death results from ischemia and hypoxia. The acidosis that accompanies ischemia denatures cellular proteins and hydrolytic enzymes. Seen with myocardial infarction, for example.

Types of tissue repair

1. Repair by regeneration
   - With regeneration, the injured tissue is repaired with the same tissue that was lost. A full return of function occurs and afterward there is little or no evidence of the injury.
   - Repair by regeneration can occur only in *labile cells* (cells that continue to divide throughout life) or *stable cells* (cells that have stopped dividing but can be induced to regenerate under appropriate conditions of injury). Examples of labile cells include those of the skin, oral cavity and bone marrow. Examples of stable cells include hepatocytes of the liver. Certain cells such as nerve cells and cardiac muscle cells are *fixed* cells and cannot undergo regeneration under any circumstances. These cell types are capable of repairing injuries through connective tissue replacement.
2. Repair by connective tissue replacement
   - Involves the replacement of functional tissue with nonfunctional connective tissue (collagen).
   - Full function does not return to the injured tissue.
   - Scar tissue remains as evidence of the injury.

Steps in tissue (wound) repair

Clean, neat wounds such as surgical incisions are said to heal by *primary intention* since they tend to heal quickly and evenly with a minimum of tissue loss. *Sutures* are used to bring the edges of wounds together to facilitate the process of healing by primary intention. Larger, open-type wounds may take considerably longer to heal and are said to heal by *secondary intention*. These larger wounds often require a large amount of tissue replacement and tend to be associated with significant scar formation. In general, tissue repair involves three stages:

1. Inflammatory stage
   - Starts with formation of a fibrin blood clot to stem bleeding from the injury.
   - Infiltration of phagocytic white blood cells occurs. Neutrophils tend to arrive first, followed by larger macrophages. The arriving macrophages produce *growth factors* that stimulate growth of epithelial cells around the wound as well as *angiogenesis* (the formation of new blood vessels).
2. Proliferative stage
   - From 1 to 3 days after the initial injury, *fibroblasts* in and around the injured tissue proliferate in response to growth factors such as *fibroblast-activating factors* produced by infiltrating macrophages. These activated fibroblasts produce the collagen that will repair the bulk of the wound. Epithelial cells at the margins of the

wound also proliferate in response to macrophage-produced growth factors. Angiogenesis is likewise occurring at this point. The soft, pink tissue that forms during this phase of wound healing is referred to as *granulation tissue.*
   - Over time, the collagen that is laid down adds mechanical strength to the repaired area. *Contraction* of the wound occurs over the course of 1 to 2 weeks, as the edges of the wound grow closer to one another.
3. Maturation and remodeling
   - Over the course of one to several months following the injury, there is continued synthesis of collagen in conjunction with removal of old collagen by *collagenase* enzymes. This *remodeling* of the collagen is designed to maximize the strength of the repair. Capillaries that were present in the repaired area begin to disappear, leaving an avascular scar. The maturation and remodeling phase of the healed wound may continue for a number of years; however, for larger wounds, the final healed scar will never have the full tensile strength that the original tissue had prior to the injury.
   - A number of factors can impair the wound healing process (see Table 1.3).

Table 1.3 Factors That Impair Wound Healing

Malnutrition
Poor blood flow and hypoxia
Impaired immune response (immunosuppressive drugs, diseases affecting immune function such as HIV and diabetes)
Infection of wound
Foreign particles in the wound
Old age (decreased immune activity, poor circulation, poor nutrition)

Keloid scars

Large, raised scars that result from oversynthesis of collagen and decreased collagen breakdown. Keloid scars are often unsightly and may extend beyond the original boundaries of the wound. A familial tendency for keloid scar formation has been observed with a greater occurrence in blacks than whites.

chapter two

Cancer

Study objectives

- List the main characteristics of benign and malignant tumors.
- Describe the nomenclature used for various types of tumors.
- Discuss tumor metastasis. How do tumors facilitate their own spread? What are some common sites of metastasis for tumors?
- Define oncogenesis. Discuss some of the theories of how it might occur. List some viruses that are oncogenic, as well as the cancers they may cause.
- What is a carcinogen? List some substances that are carcinogenic.
- List the local and systemic effects of cancer.
- Define cancer cachexia. Why might it occur?
- Describe the system by which tumors are "staged."
- What are tumor cell markers? How are they used clinically?
- Discuss the various treatment options for cancer. Include the drawbacks of each.

Introduction

Cancer is a disease that results from abnormal growth and differentiation of tissues. Cancer is the second leading cause of death in the United States (see Table 2.1). The most common sites for cancer development are the prostate, breast, lung and colon.[4] Although cancer can arise at any age, the incidence of cancer increases proportionally with increasing age.

Table 2.1 Estimated Number of New Cancer Cases for 2001 in the United States

Cancer	Male	Female
All	643,000	625,000
Oral cavity and pharynx	20,200	9,900
Digestive system	124,000	111,700
Respiratory	102,400	82,200
Breast	1,500	192,200
Genital	206,500	80,300
Urinary system	59,400	28,100
Brain	9,800	7,400
Endocrine	5,600	15,800
Lymphoma	35,000	28,600
Leukemia	17,700	13,800

Source: Adapted from the American Cancer Society 2001 Surveillance Report, www.cancer.org/eprise/main/docroot/stt/stt_0.

Cancer terminology

Tumor or *neoplasm* — A mass of tissue in which the growth rate is excessive and uncoordinated when compared with normal tissues (see Table 2.2).

Benign neoplasm — Tumor cells that tend to be clustered in a single mass and are not malignant. Benign tumors usually will not cause death unless they interfere with vital function. Specific names end with "*oma*." For example, a hepatoma is a benign tumor of the liver, whereas a hepatocarcinoma is a malignant tumor.

Table 2.2 Characteristics of Neoplasia

Benign	Malignant
Slow growth rate	Rapid growth rate
Encapsulated	Non-encapsulated
Well-differentiated cells	Undifferentiated (anaplasia)
Resemble tissue of origin	Loss of contact inhibition
Do not metastasize	Metastasize readily
	Express foreign antigens
	Abnormal gene expression

Malignant neoplasm — Tumors that have the ability to *metastasize* or break loose and spread to other areas of the body. If untreated, such tumors can cause great suffering and death. Specific examples:

Carcinoma — Malignant tumor of *epithelial cell origin.*

Sarcoma — Malignant tumor of *skeletal or connective tissue origin.*

Lymphoma — Malignant tumor of *lymphatic tissue.*

Glioma — Malignant tumor of the *glial support cells* in the central nervous system.

Metastasis — The ability of tumor cells to spread to other parts of the body and establish secondary tumors. Malignant tumor cells can break off and utilize blood vessels or lymphatic vessels to spread to other areas of the body. Tumor cells enhance their potential for metastatic spread by releasing *protease* enzymes that digest the extracellular matrix surrounding adjacent cells. Malignant tumor cells may also produce *growth factors* that stimulate the formation of new blood vessels (*angiogenesis*), which in turn support the rapid growth of tumor cells. Certain organs such as the lungs are prime locations for the formation of metastases because of the large amount of blood flow they receive from the body. The liver is also a common site of metastasis for tumors originating in the gastrointestinal tract because blood draining the intestines must first pass through the liver via the hepatic portal system. Some common sites of metastasis for various cancers are listed in Table 2.3.

Table 2.3 Common Sites of Metastasis for Selected Cancers

Breast cancer — Bones, lymph nodes (axillary), brain
Lung cancer — Many organs including liver, brain and bone
Prostate cancer — Bones, lungs, liver, endocrine glands
Colon cancer — Liver
Testicular cancer — Lungs, liver
Ovarian cancer — Peritoneum, liver, lungs, diaphragm

Theories of oncogenesis

Oncogenesis is the process by which normal cells are transformed into cancer cells.

Abnormalities of tumor suppressor/inducer genes

Several proteins produced within cells such as the *p53* protein are known to limit cellular division by regulating certain parts of the normal cell cycle.[5] The genes that code for these proteins are referred to as *anti-oncogenes* since they suppress cell growth. Failure of these anti-oncogenes may lead to the unregulated cellular division that is characteristic of cancer cells. In contrast, other groups of genes are classified as *proto-oncogenes* since they produce proteins and substances that enhance cellular growth and proliferation.

Excessive activity of these genes (or a lack of their regulation) may likewise cause excessive cellular division and growth.

Mutation of DNA

Numerous chemical, physical and biologic agents have been shown to be *carcinogenic*, meaning they can induce the formation of cancers (see Table 2.4). Many of these agents can damage cellular DNA, either directly or through the production of toxic intermediates such as free radicals. Certain viruses are also *oncogenic* in that they may induce mutations in host cell DNA or alter rates of cellular transcription (see Table 2.5). Mutations of cellular DNA can lead to the formation of cells with abnormal growth and differentiation patterns.

Table 2.4 Possible Cancer-Causing Agents

Chemicals — Many such as benzene, vinyl chloride, cigarette smoke, aromatic hydrocarbons
Radiation, radon gas, radioactive materials, ultraviolet radiation
Occupational exposure — Asbestos, coal dust, uranium, solvents
Oncogenic viruses
Dietary factors — High-fat diet, excessive alcohol intake, nitrosamine preservatives, grilled or charred foods
Hormones — Estrogens, progesterone

Table 2.5 Oncogenic Viruses in Humans

A number of DNA and RNA viruses have been shown to be "oncogenic," meaning they can cause cancers in the hosts they infect.
Human Papillomavirus — Cervical carcinoma
Hepatitis B Virus — Liver cancer
Epstein–Barr Virus — Burkitt's lymphoma, nasopharyngeal cancer
HIV Virus — Kaposi's sarcoma

Hereditary

A genetic predisposition has been observed for a number of cancers including colon cancer, breast cancer, retinoblastoma and certain forms of leukemia and lymphoma. A great deal of recent research has focused on identifying certain genetic markers in individuals that might pinpoint them as at risk for the development of certain types of cancer.[6]

Manifestations of cancer

Many cancers may be asymptomatic in the early stages. As the tumors continue to grow, they affect local tissues as well as the overall body.

1. Local effects of cancer
   - Compression of blood vessels

- Ischemia
- Pain
- Bleeding
- Infection
- Altered tissue function

2. Systemic effects of cancer
   - Fatigue
   - *Cachexia* (see Cachexia box)
   - Bleeding and hemorrhage
   - Anemia due to chronic bleeding or bone marrow destruction; this anemia may be exacerbated by chemotherapy
   - Altered organ function
   - Abnormal hormone production from an affected gland or directly from certain types of hormone-producing tumors

---

Cachexia

A complex syndrome characterized by anorexia, weight loss and lean body (muscle) wasting seen in a significant percent of patients with cancer and AIDS. A number of metabolic abnormalities have been demonstrated in patients with cachexia that lead to poor utilization of nutrients and overall malnutrition. A key factor in cachexia appears to be the production of *cytokines* such as *tumor necrosis factor* and *interleukins* in response to the presence of cancer. These substances are produced by many cells within the body and appear to be protective against bacterial and viral infections as well as malignant cells. Unfortunately, these substances also appear to be responsible for many of the effects of cachexia including anorexia and lean body wasting.[7]

Tumor staging

Tumors are classified or "staged" based upon the "TNM" system that includes a description of tumor size (T), involvement of lymph nodes (N) and metastasis (M). The TNM system for staging tumors is explained in Table 2.6.

Cancer detection

Tumor cell markers (see Table 2.7)

- Substances produced by or found on the surface of tumor cells.
- Tumor cell markers may be used clinically to screen for the presence of tumor cells in the body.

Table 2.6 Staging of Tumors

T — Primary tumor (Is there a tumor and if so how big is it?)
TX — Primary tumor cannot be assessed
TO — No evidence of primary tumor
Tis — Carcinoma *in situ*
T1–T4 — Increasing size of tumor
N — Involvement of lymph nodes (Has the tumor spread to the lymph nodes?)
NX — Regional lymph nodes cannot be assessed
NO — No evidence that the tumor has metastasized to lymph nodes in the region of the primary tumor
N1–N3 — Progressive involvement of regional lymph nodes
M — Distant metastasis (Has the tumor spread to distant sites in the body?)
Mx — Distant metastasis cannot be assessed
MO — No evidence of distant metastasis
M1–M4 — Single or multiple sites of metastasis have been located

Table 2.7 Examples of Tumor Cell Markers

α-Fetopotein
Secreted by embryonic liver cells
High levels seen in liver, ovarian and testicular cancer
May also be observed with viral hepatitis
Prostate-specific antigen (PSA)
Markedly increased in prostatic cancer
Slightly elevated in benign prostatic hypertrophy
CA 15-3
Elevated in breast cancer
High levels often indicate advanced or metastatic breast cancer
May be elevated in benign breast disease or liver disease
CA 19-9
Elevated in cancers of the gastrointestinal tract and pancreas
May also be elevated in gallbladder disease and pancreatitis
CA 27-29
Elevated in breast cancer as well as a number of other cancers
May also be elevated in benign breast disease as well as disease of the kidney and liver
CA 125
Elevated in ovarian cancer
May be elevated in pregnancy and with pelvic inflammatory disease
Human chorionic gonadotrophin
Used as a marker for a number of different cancers
Elevated in pregnancy

- Drawbacks to the use of tumor markers in cancer diagnosis include that they may not be specific for a certain type of cancer and that by the time tumor cell markers are detected, the particular cancer may be well progressed. In addition, certain noncancerous conditions may also be associated with the appearance of some of these markers in the blood.

Visualization

- Radiography, computer tomography (CT scans), magnetic resonance imaging
- *Endoscopy* may also be utilized to visually detect tumors in the bronchi and gastrointestinal tract
- Identifies the presence of a tumor or tumors; can also be used to evaluate metastasis

Biopsy

- Removal of a piece of suspect tissue for detailed histologic or histochemical analysis
- May be accomplished surgically, by a needle biopsy, by scraping cells from a surface (Pap smear) or by endoscopic biopsy

Rationale for therapy

Cancer treatment can be multifaceted and may include surgical removal of tumors, as well as chemotherapy and/or radiation therapy to kill or arrest rapidly growing tumor cells. A number of immune-based treatments are currently under investigation as alternatives to toxic chemotherapy and radiation therapy. Treatment with specific hormones has also been shown to inhibit the growth of certain types of cancers.

Treatment of cancer

Surgical removal

If accessible, tumors should be surgically removed. Often accompanied by chemotherapy or radiation therapy to kill any cancer cells that are not removed or have metastasized.

Chemotherapy

Drugs used for chemotherapy of cancer fall into several categories (see Table 2.8).

Hormonal therapy

Sex hormones are routinely used to inhibit tumor growth in breast, prostate and uterine cancer. The estrogen inhibitor *tamoxifen* has also been shown to be effective in the treatment of breast cancer and may eventually be used as a prophylactic agent in women who are at a high risk for developing breast cancer. The androgen inhibitor *flutamide* has also been approved for treatment of prostate cancer.

Table 2.8 Chemotherapy Drugs

Alkylating agents and nitrosureas (examples: cyclophosphamide, carmustine)
Cytotoxic to cancer cells due to alkylation of cancer cell DNA
Major toxicities include nausea and vomiting, and bone marrow suppression
Antimetabolites (examples: methotrexate, fluorouracil)
Inhibit synthesis of essential nucleotides and nucleic acids in cancer cells
Major toxicities include myelosuppression, nausea, vomiting, oral and gastrointestinal ulceration
Plant alkaloids (examples: vinblastine, vincristine)
Disrupt mitosis in cancer cells by interfering with formation of the mitotic spindle
Numerous toxicities including cardiotoxicity, bone marrow depression, neurologic and muscle effects as well as alopecia
Antibiotics (examples: doxorubicin, bleomycin)
Bind directly to cancer cell DNA to block the formation of new RNA or DNA
Major toxicities include bone marrow suppression, alopecia

Radiation therapy

Radiation therapy utilizes ionizing or particle beam radiation to destroy cancer cells that are highly mitotic and most susceptible to the lethal effects of radiation. Radiation therapy can have a number of localized and systemic side effects including alopecia, diarrhea, tissue irritation and organ inflammation.

Immune-based therapies

"Biologic response modifiers" such as *interferons, immunomodulators, tumor antigens* and *lymphokines/cytokines* are being investigated as means of enhancing the immune system response of individuals with cancer. *Monoclonal antibodies* have also been studied as a highly specific means of delivering chemotherapeutic drugs directly to and only to cancer cells.

chapter three

Disorders of hemostasis and coagulation

Study objectives

- List and describe the steps involved in hemostasis.
- Compare and contrast the intrinsic and extrinsic pathways of blood clotting.
- Discuss the various genetic conditions that lead to abnormal bleeding.
- Describe the various means by which acquired bleeding disorders might occur.
- List drugs that might impair hemostasis and blood clotting.
- List conditions that might lead to hypercoagulability.

Introduction

Hemostasis is a term that refers to the stoppage of blood flow. Normal hemostasis involves a series of reactions designed to arrest bleeding from a site of injury through formation of a platelet plug and fibrin clot. *Coagulation* is the process by which blood is converted from the liquid to the solid state, namely, the fibrin clot. Blood coagulation is an essential component of hemostasis. When the process of hemostasis becomes impaired, the ability to effectively stop bleeding is lost. In contrast, should the mechanisms involved in hemostasis and blood coagulation become overly active, unwanted clots may form within the blood vessels or tissues.

Steps in hemostasis

The process of hemostasis may be divided into four key steps:

1. Vascular spasm
2. Formation of a platelet plug
3. Activation of blood coagulation cascade
4. Formation of a fibrin clot

Vascular spasm

- Vasoconstriction occurs immediately following injury to a blood vessel wall to limit blood flow out of the vessel.
- A key mediator of the vasoconstriction appears to be *thromboxane* A_2, which is released both from circulating platelets in the area of injury and the damaged endothelial cells themselves.

Formation of platelet plug

- Platelets *aggregate* at the site of injury. The platelet plug is able to seal small openings in blood vessel walls to stop minor bleeding.
- Platelets are attracted to the area of injury, and exposure to substances at the site of injury such as antigens, collagen and bacterial toxins causes platelets to change shape and become "sticky." These sticky platelets now adhere to exposed collagen on the basement membranes of injured blood vessels. This process is called *adhesion*.
- Proper adhesion of platelets requires the release of a protein from vascular endothelial cells called *von Willebrand's factor*. This protein is essential for allowing platelets to adhere to collagen as well as to one another.
- Once platelets have undergone the process of adhesion, substances such as thrombin, thromboxane A_2 and ADP lead to further platelet *activation*. Activated platelets now release the contents of their

internal granules, which include substances such as ADP, fibrinogen, thrombin, thromboxane A_2 and von Willebrand's factor, which induce the *aggregation* of additional platelets at the injury site.

Activation of blood coagulation cascades

- Blood coagulation is the process in which *fibrin* protein strands wrap around the platelet plug to form an insoluble clot.
- The process of blood coagulation occurs through two separate, but related pathways called the *intrinsic coagulation pathway* and the *extrinsic coagulation pathway* (see Figure 3.1).

Intrinsic pathway

- Initiated by protein factors found circulating in the blood.
- Activation of initial clotting factor *XII* (Hageman factor) occurs through contact with exposed collagen or damaged endothelium.

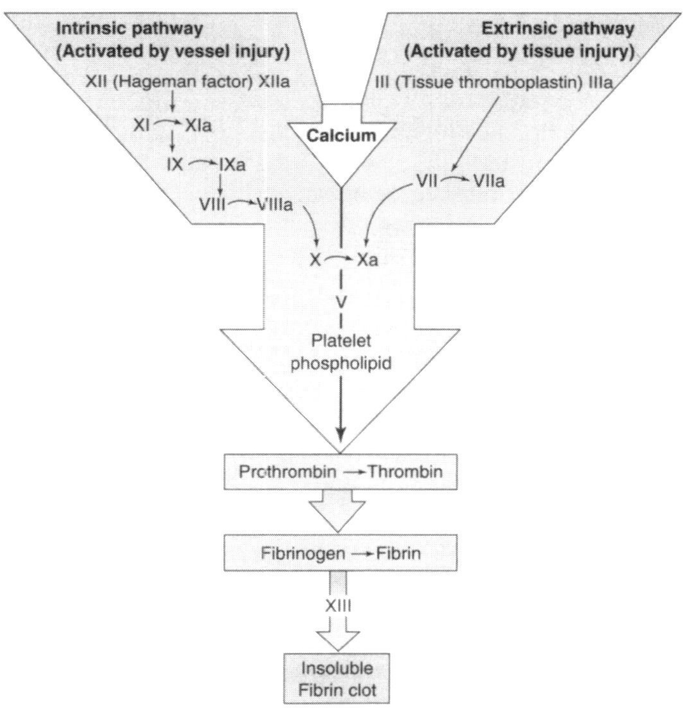

Figure 3.1 Coagulation pathways. (From Porth, C.M., *Pathophysiology: Concepts of Altered Health States*, 5th ed., Lippincott, Philadelphia, 1998. With permission.)

Extrinsic pathway

- Initiated by protein factors located in the tissues.
- Activation of extrinsic pathway occurs when factor *III* (thromboplastin) is released from tissues to activate clotting factor *VII*.

Both *intrinsic* and *extrinsic* pathways converge at clotting factor *X*, which originates both in plasma and tissues. The final common sequence in both pathways involves a complex that includes activated factor *X*, factor *V*, platelet phospholipids and Ca^{2+} that catalyzes the conversion of the serum protein *prothrombin* to *thrombin*. In turn, thrombin converts plasma *fibrinogen* to *fibrin*, the substance that polymerizes to form the insoluble clot. A final factor *(XIII)*, called *clot-stabilizing factor*, is released by platelets trapped in the platelet plug and stimulates polymerization and cross-linking of fibrin strands.

Formation of fibrin clot

Clot retraction

Retraction is a process that occurs once the fibrin clot has formed. It involves contraction and shrinkage of the fibrin strands and is induced by continued release of factor *XIII* from platelets. Clot retraction serves to pull the edges of the damaged blood vessel together to facilitate the repair process.

Fibrinolysis (clot dissolution)

Once the damaged blood vessel is repaired, the fibrin clot is no longer needed and must be removed from the blood vessel lining. This process of *fibrinolysis* or *clot dissolution* is accomplished by the enzyme *plasmin* that digests the fibrin strands of the clot as well as several clotting factors. Plasmin travels in circulation as the inactive pro-enzyme *plasminogen*. Factors produced by the liver and vascular endothelium called *plasminogen activators* — tissue-type plasminogen activator (t-PA) and urokinase-type plasminogen activator (u-PA) — convert the pro-enzyme plasminogen to the active fibrinolytic enzyme plasmin. The activity of plasmin is in turn regulated by the inhibitory enzyme *α_2-plasmin inhibitor*, which rapidly inactivates it.

Conditions leading to decreased coagulation

Genetic defects

1. Hemophilia
2. von Willebrand's disease

Hemophilia

Hemophilia is caused by a genetic deficiency or lack of certain clotting factors. Three distinct types of hemophilia have been identified.

Type A hemophilia

- Most common form (80% or more)
- X-linked recessive disorder
- Results from a deficiency of clotting factor VIII

Type B hemophilia (Christmas disease)

- Second most common form of hemophilia (10 to 15%)
- X-linked autosomal recessive disorder
- Results from a deficiency of clotting factor IX

Type C hemophilia (Rosenthal's disease)

- Least common of all hemophilia cases (<5%)
- Results from a deficiency of clotting factor XI
- Autosomal recessive disorder

Manifestations of hemophilia

- May present as a mild, moderate or severe bleeding disorder depending on the activity of the clotting factors
- Excessive bleeding with trauma or surgery
- Bleeding into soft tissues, muscles and joints

Treatment of hemophilia

- Avoidance of injury, prevention of bleeding
- Replacement with recombinant clotting factors

There was a significant incidence of HIV and hepatitis C in patients with hemophilia before the advent of recombinant clotting factors because these factors were previously derived from donor blood.

von Willebrand's disease

- Most common hereditary bleeding disorder
- Caused by a genetic lack of von Willebrand's factor
- Causes a reduction in platelet adhesion
- Symptoms may include excessive bruising and mild to moderate bleeding
- Bleeding may occur from gums, nose, gastrointestinal tract; blood flow during menstruation may be especially heavy

Treatment of von Willebrand's disease

- Infusion of von Willebrand's factor
- *Desmopressin acetate* — A vasopressin analogue that increases the activity of factor VIII and may stimulate production of von Willebrand's factor by endothelial cells

Autoimmune defects

Idiopathic thrombocytopenia purpura

- Most commonly occurs in children and adolescents following a viral infection.
- Autoimmune disorder in which antibodies bind to platelets in circulation. Antibody-bound platelets are now more susceptible to destruction in the spleen. Enlargement of the spleen may result.
- Patients may present with abnormal bruising and bleeding.
- A chronic, lifelong form of the disorder may also occur with lesser incidence.
- Treatment may include immunosuppressing drugs like corticosteroids, and possible splenectomy for the chronic form.

Thrombocytopenia

Thrombocytopenia is defined as any condition in which the platelet count is abnormally low ($<100{,}000/mm^3$). Decreased platelet production can accompany conditions in which bone marrow function is altered, such as:

- Cancer
- Aplastic anemia
- Drug or chemical-induced destruction of platelets
- Radiation exposure
- Infection, HIV
- Deficiency of vitamin B_{12}, folic acid
- Autoimmune destruction

Acquired deficiencies

Vitamin K deficiency

- Vitamin K is essential for synthesis of factors II, VII, IX and X.
- It must be obtained from the diet via bacterial metabolism.
- Conditions that may lead to vitamin K deficiency include intestinal malabsorption or destruction of intestinal flora by antibiotics.
- Treatment may include infusion of deficient factors and replacement of parenteral vitamin K.

Liver disease

Because the clotting factors are synthesized by the liver, any disease or condition that alters liver function may lead to defective production of clotting factors. Diseases that can alter the function of the liver include the following:

- Hepatitis
- Cirrhosis
- Liver cancer
- Liver failure

Drug-induced alterations in hemostasis and coagulation

A number of pharmacologic agents can impair blood clotting by inhibiting platelet function. These agents include the *nonsteroidal anti-inflammatories, β-lactam antibiotics,* certain *antidepressants* and a number of *cardiovascular drugs.* Other drugs can interfere with the action of coagulation factors and may be used therapeutically as *anticoagulants* (see Table 3.1).

Table 3.1 Anticoagulant Drugs

Warfarin
Used orally
Acts by preventing the reduction of *vitamin K,* an essential cofactor in the formation of clotting factors II, VII, IX and X
Heparin
Used only by injection
A "family" of related compounds with molecular weights of 3000 to 40,000
Enhances the actions of the natural anticoagulant *antithrombin III*
Major unwanted effects of both oral and injected anticoagulant drugs are unwanted bleeding and possible hemorrhage

Conditions leading to increased blood coagulation

Individuals with hypercoagulability are at increased risk for venous thrombus and emboli. Conditions that can cause hypercoagulability include the following:

- Inherited disorders of coagulation
- Polycythemia
- Obesity
- Prolonged bed rest
- Cancer
- Venous stasis
- Sepsis
- Trauma or surgery

chapter four

Alterations in hematologic function and oxygen transport

Study objectives

- List the major components of blood.
- Outline the process of erythropoiesis and discuss the role of hypoxia and erythropoietin.
- Compare and contrast the various types of anemia in terms of etiology and major manifestations.
- Describe how anemia may be classified by size and color of red blood cells.
- Define polycythemia.

Introduction

Blood is composed of two main components: a liquid portion called *plasma* and a cellular portion containing red blood cells (*erythrocytes),* white blood cells (*leukocytes*) and platelets (*thrombocytes*). Blood serves a number of important functions in the human body such as transport of oxygen, nutrients and ions while acting as a buffer between cells and the environment. The total blood volume in a 70-kg man is approximately 5 L. Table 4.1 summarizes the major components of whole blood.

Table 4.1 Components of Whole Blood

Plasma	Cells
Water (97%)	Red blood cells
Ions	White blood cells
Organics	Platelets
Protein	
Sugars	
Amino acids	
Lipids	
Trace elements	
Dissolved gases	

Hematopoiesis

The process by which blood cells are formed is called *hematopoiesis* (see Figure 4.1). All of the cellular components in blood are derived from a common precursor called a *stem cell*. In the maturing fetus, early production of erythrocytes takes place in developing blood vessels. As gestation continues, the production of both red and white blood cells shifts to the fetal liver and spleen and eventually is localized primarily in the bone marrow. Hematopoiesis continues in the bone marrow after birth and is a lifelong process. A number of growth factors and cytokines are involved in regulating the process of hematopoiesis. A major regulator of red blood cell production is the hormone *erythropoietin* that is produced by the adult kidney. Erythropoietin is a glycoprotein released by cells of the kidney in response to the presence of *hypoxia*. The erythropoietin that is produced acts directly on stem cells in the bone marrow to promote the proliferation, maturation and release of new erythrocytes. The mature red blood cells that form are biconcave in structure and lack a nucleus. The unique shape of the mature erythrocyte maximizes surface area and facilitates diffusion of oxygen across the cell membrane. Because red blood cells do not contain mitochondria, they rely primarily on glycolysis to meet their metabolic needs. The cell membranes of normal red blood cells must be strong enough to survive transport under high pressure yet be flexible enough to fit through narrow and winding capillaries. A protein *cytoskeleton* provides a framework of support to the red blood cell membrane.

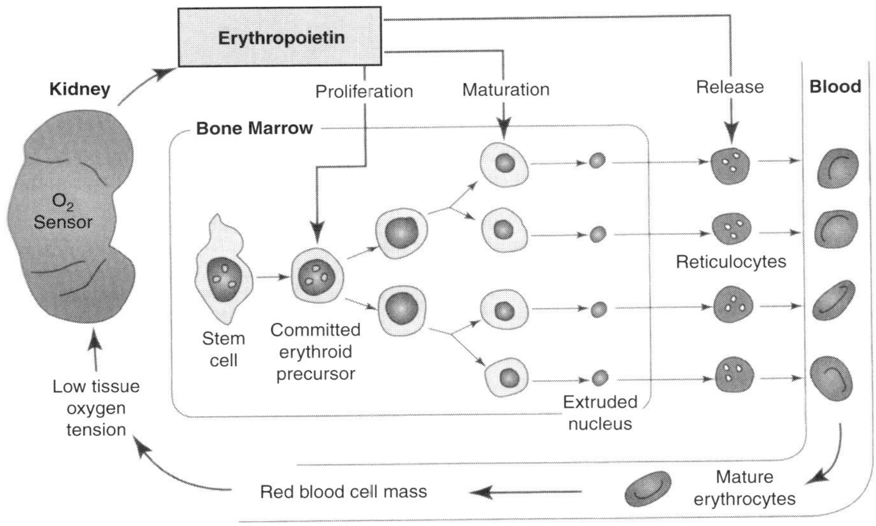

Figure 4.1 Hematopoiesis. The role of enthropoietin and hypoxia. (From Porth, C.M., *Pathophysiology: Concepts of Altered Health States*, 5th ed., Lippincott, Philadelphia, 1998. With permission.)

Table 4.2 Analysis of Blood Cells

A sample of blood is collected by venipuncture. Tests performed may include:

Complete blood count (CBC) — A count of red blood cells, white blood cells and platelets
White blood cell differential count — Determines the percent of each type of white cell present in the blood
Mean corpuscular hemoglobin concentration (MCHC) — Measure of the amount of hemoglobin in each red blood cell
Mean corpuscular volume (MCV) — Measure of the size or volume of red blood cells
Hematocrit — The volume of red blood cells expressed as a fraction of the total volume of the blood
Morphologic examination — To detect changes in blood cell shape or size
Erythrocyte sedimentation rate — The rate at which red blood cells settle out of suspension; changes with alterations in plasma protein concentration, chronic infection and malignancy

The function of red blood cells is to transport oxygen to tissues. This is accomplished by the intracellular protein *hemoglobin*. The quaternary hemoglobin protein is composed of two α and two β subunits. Each of the subunits contains a central iron containing protein called a *heme* protein. It is the iron atom in the heme protein that binds to molecular oxygen. As a result of the four iron-containing heme groups, each molecule of hemoglobin can carry four atoms of oxygen.

Anemia

Anemia is a condition in which there is a reduced number of red blood cells or decreased concentration of hemoglobin in those cells or both. Anemia is often a manifestation of some disease process or abnormality within the body. Although there are many causes of anemia, the actual mechanism by which the anemia results is generally due to (1) excess loss or destruction of red blood cells and (2) reduced or defective production of red blood cells. Anemias may be classified according to cause or effect on red cell morphology (see Table 4.3).

General manifestations of anemia

A major feature of anemia is a reduced capacity for the transport of oxygen to tissues. This reduced oxygen delivery can result in the following:

- Ischemia
- Fatigability
- Breathlessness upon exertion
- Exercise intolerance
- Pallor
- Increased susceptibility to infection

Types of anemia

Hemolytic anemia

Anemia that results from excess destruction of red blood cells (*hemolysis*). Factors that may cause hemolysis include the following:

- Autoimmune destruction of red blood cells
- Certain drugs (example: quinine) or toxins
- Cancers such as lymphoma and leukemia

Table 4.3 Classification of Anemia Based on Red Cell Morphology

Size changes
Normocytic anemia — RBC size is unchanged
Example: Blood loss anemia
Macrocytic anemia — RBC size is increased
Example: B_{12}/folic acid deficiency anemia
Microcytic anemia — RBC size is reduced
Example: Iron deficiency anemia
Color changes (due to altered hemoglobin content)
Normochromic — Normal hemoglobin concentration
Hypochromic — Reduced hemoglobin concentration
Example: Iron deficiency anemia may be classified as a microcytic, hypochromic anemia as both red blood cell size and hemoglobin content are reduced

- Rheumatoid arthritis
- Certain viral infections (parvovirus)
- Parasitic infections (malaria)

Blood loss anemia

Anemia that results from acute blood loss. With acute loss of large amounts of blood, shock is the major concern. With chronic loss of smaller amounts of blood, iron deficiency is a chief concern. Causes of acute and chronic blood loss may include the following:

- Trauma and hemorrhage
- Malignancy
- Peptic ulcers

Iron-deficiency anemia

Iron-deficiency anemia is a major cause of anemia worldwide. It can occur as a result of iron-deficient diets. Vegetarians are at particular risk for iron deficiency as are menstruating or pregnant women due to increased requirement for iron. Iron-deficiency anemia may also result from poor absorption of iron from the intestine or persistent blood loss (e.g., ulcers, neoplasia). Because iron is the functional component of hemoglobin, lack of available iron will result in a decreased hemoglobin synthesis and subsequent impairment of red blood cell oxygen-carrying capacity.

Cobalamin-deficiency or folate-deficiency anemia

Cobalamin (vitamin B_{12}) and folic acid are essential nutrients required for DNA synthesis and red cell maturation, respectively. Deficiency of these nutrients will lead to the formation of red blood cells that are of abnormal shape with shortened life spans due to weakened cell membranes. One important cause of vitamin B_{12} deficiency is *pernicious anemia* that results from a lack of *intrinsic factor* production by the gastric mucosa. Intrinsic factor is required for normal absorption of vitamin B_{12} from the intestine. Any intestinal abnormalities (e.g., neoplasia, inflammation) that interfere with the production of intrinsic factor can lead to vitamin B_{12} deficiency. Folic acid deficiency most commonly results from poor diet, malnutrition or intestinal malabsorption.

Inherited anemia

Anemia may also result from genetic defects in red blood cell structure or function. Two common genetic disorders of erythrocytes are *sickle cell anemia* and *thalassemia*. Both of these disorders result from abnormal or absent genes for the production of hemoglobin.

Sickle cell disease

Sickle cell disease is a group of autosomal recessive disorders characterized by abnormal hemoglobin production. In the United States the highest prevalence of sickle cell disease is in blacks with a reported incidence of approximately 1 in 500 births. Sickle cell disease has several patterns of inheritance that determine the severity of the disease in afflicted individuals. In the *homozygous* form of the disease, most of the hemoglobin formed is defective and the clinical presentation is most severe. With the *heterozygous* form of the disease, less than half of the red cell hemoglobin is affected and the presentation is significantly milder. Individuals may also inherit the *sickle cell trait* and be carriers of the defective hemoglobin gene without significant clinical manifestations.

Manifestations of sickle cell disease: The abnormal hemoglobin formed in sickle cell disease results from a substitution mutation of a single amino acid. This mutation causes the deoxygenated hemoglobin to clump and become abnormally rigid. The rigidity of the defective hemoglobin deforms the pliable red blood cell membrane and causes erythrocytes to take on "sickled" or half-moon appearance. The degree of sickling that occurs is determined by the amount of abnormal hemoglobin within the red blood cell and only occurs when the abnormal hemoglobin is deoxygenated. As a result of their elongated shape and rigidity, affected blood cells do not pass easily through narrow blood vessels. *Hemolysis* of sickled red blood cells is also common. The *spleen* is a major site of red cell hemolysis since the blood vessels found within this organ are narrow and convoluted. As a result of the sluggish blood flow, many tissues and organs of the body are eventually affected by this disorder. Specific manifestations may include the following:

- Impaired oxygen-carrying capacity resulting in fatigue, pallor
- Occlusion of blood vessels leading to ischemia, hypoxia, pain
- Organ damage
- Splenomegaly due to increased destruction of red blood cells in this organ
- Jaundice as a result of increased amounts of hemoglobin released into circulation (see Jaundice box)
- Increased risk of infection and possible septicemia due to stagnation of blood

---

Jaundice

Jaundice occurs when there is an excess of *bilirubin* in the blood. Bilirubin is a breakdown product of hemoglobin that is excreted into the bile. In *hemolytic anemia* excess rates of red blood cell destruction lead to the production of bilirubin at rates faster than it can be eliminated from the liver and as a result bilirubin backs up into the blood. Bilirubin is pigmented and taints the skin and whites of the eyes with a characteristic yellowish tinge that is indicative of jaundice.

Thalassemia

Thalassemia is a genetic disorder characterized by absent or defective production of hemoglobin α or β chains. As with sickle cell anemia, afflicted individuals may be *heterozygous* for the trait and have a milder presentation of the disease or *homozygous* and have a more severe form of the disorder. The β form of thalassemia (defective formation of β hemoglobin chains) is most common in individuals from Mediterranean populations, whereas the α form of thalassemia (defective formation of α hemoglobin chains) occurs mostly in Asians. Both the α and β forms of thalassemia are common in blacks.

Manifestations of thalassemia

In heterozygous individuals enough normal hemoglobin is usually synthesized to prevent significant anemia. In these individuals symptoms of anemia may appear only with exercise or physiologic stress. Homozygous individuals are often dependent on frequent transfusions to treat the resulting severe anemia. Children affected with the homozygous form may suffer severe growth retardation. The widespread *hypoxia* that can result from impaired oxygen-carrying capacity leads to *erythropoietin-induced* increases in hematopoiesis that can eventually affect the structure of the long bones. Severe anemia may also lead to congestive heart failure and marked hepatosplenomegaly. Excessive hemolysis of red blood cells may occur in severe forms of the disease due to overproduction of the normal hemoglobin subunit. Iron deposits from increased absorption and frequent transfusions may injure the liver and heart as well.

Treatment of sickle cell anemia and thalassemia

Individuals with inherited anemia should avoid physiologic stresses that might exacerbate hypoxia. Infections should be avoided and promptly treated if they occur to prevent a possible hypoxic crisis. Proper immunizations and vaccinations should be administered to lessen the chance of infection. Frequent transfusions of normal erythrocytes are commonly used in individuals with severe forms of inherited anemia during periods of crisis. These individuals are at risk for iron accumulation as well as contracting blood-borne pathogens such as hepatitis and HIV from improperly screened blood. Bone marrow transplant may be utilized effectively to cure patients with genetic anemias; however, the procedure carries considerable risk of its own.[8]

Aplastic anemia

Aplastic anemia results from a lack of red blood cell production by the bone marrow. If erythrocyte stem cell precursors are lacking or destroyed, the process of erythropoiesis will be severely impaired. Aplastic anemia may result from a congenital defect in stem cell production or can be caused by exposure to agents that damage the bone marrow such as solvents,

Table 4.4 Possible Causes of Aplastic Anemia

Radiation
Chemicals (organic solvents, heavy metals)
Chemotherapy drugs
Certain antibiotics (chloramphenicol)
HIV infection
Toxins

radiation, infection, chemotherapeutic drugs and certain antibiotics (see Table 4.4). Drug-induced aplastic anemia is usually a dose-dependent phenomenon. The clinical manifestations of aplastic anemia will depend on the extent to which hematopoiesis is impaired. General symptoms of anemia such as pallor, fatigue and lethargy can occur initially. Bleeding in the skin and from the nose, mouth and body orifices may also occur from a lack of platelet production by the abnormal bone marrow. Increased susceptibility to infection is also seen as a result of diminished white blood cell production. The underlying cause of the aplastic anemia needs to be identified and further exposure prevented. Treatment should also include avoidance of physiologic stresses and infection. Transfusions are effective for temporarily improving oxygen-carrying capacity. In severe cases, bone marrow transplant may offer a cure.

Polycythemia

Polycythemia is a disorder in which the number of red blood cells in circulation is greatly increased. There are two categories of polycythemia: *relative* and *primary*. *Relative polycythemia* results from an increase in the concentration of red blood cells due to a loss of plasma volume. In contrast, *primary polycythemia* (*polycythemia vera*) is caused by excessive proliferation of bone marrow stem cells. Polycythemia vera is a rare neoplastic disorder that occurs in men between the ages of 40 and 60. A secondary form of polycythemia may occur from excess *erythropoietin* production as a physiologic response to hypoxia. Secondary polycythemia may be seen in individuals living at high altitudes, in chronic smokers or in people with chronic obstructive pulmonary disease.

Manifestations

- Increased blood volume and viscosity
- Increased risk of thrombus
- Occlusion of small blood vessels
- Hepatosplenomegaly from pooling of blood
- Impaired blood flow to tissues (ischemia)

Treatment

- Increasing fluid volume in relative polycythemia
- Periodic removal of blood to reduce viscosity and volume in primary polycythemia
- Chemotherapy or radiation to suppress activity of bone marrow stem cells in polycythemia vera

chapter five

Immune response and inflammation

Study objectives

- List the three lines of defense the body has against foreign invaders. What components of the immune system are involved in each?
- Define the following terms: antigen, epitope, hapten, MHC I, MHC II.
- Discuss the role of monocytes and macrophages in the overall immune response. What are fixed macrophages?
- List the various types and subtypes of lymphocytes. Describe the role of each of these specific cells in the immune response.
- List the various types of antibodies found in the human body. Describe the main functions of each.
- What are natural killer cells? How do they differ from T cells and B cells?
- List some examples of cytokines along with their general actions on immune function.
- What is the complement system? How does it help protect the body against foreign invaders?
- List the five cardinal signs of inflammation. Why does each occur?
- Compare and contrast the vascular response phase of the inflammatory reaction with the cellular response phase. What is the importance of each of these phases?
- Discuss the four types of hypersensitivity reactions that can occur. Give examples of when each might occur.
- Define anaphylaxis. List the symptoms that accompany it.

Introduction

The human immune system is designed to protect the body against foreign substances, bacteria and viruses as well as any abnormal cells that might arise within the body itself. The immune component is only one portion of an overall host defense system that includes physical and chemical barriers to infection as well as biologic and cellular response mechanisms. Some of these "layers" of host cell defense are very general and designed to stop any and all foreign organisms, whereas others are highly specific for certain organisms. The first line of defense against invading microorganisms involves the physical barriers presented by the skin on the body surfaces and the mucous membranes that protect openings into the body. These mucous membranes are covered by secretions such as sticky mucus that can trap invading organisms. Digestive enzymes such as *lysozymes* are often found within mucous membrane secretions and provide a chemical barrier to infections. Organisms that are able to penetrate this first line of defense must now face circulating *phagocytic* white blood cells, antimicrobial substances and *natural killer cells,* all of which attack invading organisms in a nonspecific manner. In addition, the entry of these foreign organisms into the body will trigger a significant inflammatory response and possibly fever, both of which are also protective. In addition to the above nonspecific defense mechanisms, specialized cells called *lymphocytes* and antimicrobial proteins called *antibodies* can attack foreign organisms in a highly specific manner.

Components of the immune system

Antigens

- An antigen is any substance that can induce an immune response.
- Specific molecules on bacteria, viruses, pollen, plants, insect venom and transplant tissue can all act as antigens. The specific region of the antigen molecule that initiates the immune response is called the *epitope*.
- The most powerful antigens tend to be large and complex macromolecules and are most often proteins and sugars.
- A *hapten* is a small-molecular-weight molecule that can only trigger an immune response if bound to a larger antigenic macromolecule called a *carrier*.

Major histocompatability complex (MHC)

- A group of unique glycoproteins found on the surface of cells.
- Each person has a unique MHC.

- MHC was originally called *human leukocyte antigen* because it was first identified on the surface of human white blood cells (leukocytes).
- Two distinct types of MHC are found on cells: MHC I and MHC II.

MHC I

- Found on the surface of nearly all nucleated cells within the body.
- Serve as markers of "self" for the immune system. Identify cells as being normal and belonging in the body.
- Foreign organisms like viruses will often express some of their foreign antigens on the MHC I of the cells they infect. This change in MHC I signals cells of the immune system that a particular cell has been infected and is no longer "normal."

MHC II

- Found primarily on the surfaces of macrophages and other immune cells.
- Can be used by immune cells to present foreign antigens to other immune cells.

Monocytes and macrophages

- Monocytes are produced in the bone marrow and released into circulation. Monocytes migrate into tissues during injury. In the injured tissues, monocytes change shape and mature into macrophages.
- Macrophages are phagocytic cells that engulf and destroy foreign cells, particles and debris.
- When macrophages engulf a foreign organism or particle, they take the antigenic portion of what they have digested and present it on their own cell surface using their MHC II. Macrophages that exhibit foreign antigens on the MHC II are called *antigen-presenting cells* (APC). The antigen presented on the surface of the macrophages may be recognized by specific lymphocytes called *helper T cells* (see below) that, in turn, will activate other lymphocytes to attack and destroy any foreign organisms displaying that particular antigen.
- Macrophages also produce *cytokines* such as *interleukin-1* (IL-1) that enhance the inflammatory reaction.

Lymphocytes

- Derived from stem cells in the bone marrow.
- Make up 20 to 25% of all white blood cells (leukocytes).
- Two distinct types of leukocytes are found in the human body: *T lymphocytes* and *B lymphocytes*.

T lymphocytes (T cells)

- 70% of all lymphocytes.
- Produced in the bone marrow but mature in the *thymus gland.*
- Function in *cell-mediated immunity.*
- Aid in the production of antibodies.
- Two distinct subsets of T lymphocytes are present: *helper T cells* and *cytotoxic T cells.*

Helper T cells

- Express a unique protein group on their surface called *CD4.* CD stands for "cluster of differentiation" and is a means of specifically identifying different lymphocytes.
- Helper T cells are activated when they encounter foreign antigens presented on the surface of antigen-presenting cells such as macrophages.
- Once activated, helper T cells produce cytokines that stimulate the activity of macrophages, *cytotoxic T cells* and *natural killer cells* (see Figure 5.1).
- Helper T cells interact with *B lymphocytes* to stimulate their differentiation and eventual production of antibodies.

Cytotoxic T cells

- Express CD8 protein on their cell surface.
- Cytotoxic T cells are "activated" by cytokines from helper T cells.
- Activated cytotoxic T cells recognize and bind to foreign antigen presented on MHC I of infected cells.
- Cytotoxic T cells directly destroy any infected host cells they encounter by releasing *cytotoxic cytokines, cytolytic enzymes* and proteins called *perforins* that perforate and destroy the infected cell.

B lymphocytes (B cells)

- Responsible for *humoral-mediated immunity.*
- When B lymphocytes encounter a foreign antigen, they bind to it and, under the influence of cytokines released by helper T cells, mature into *plasma cells* that produce antibodies.
- A small subpopulation of activated B lymphocytes will differentiate into *memory B cells* that persist in the body for long periods of time and are capable of recognizing and rapidly responding to the same antigen if it encounters it at a later date.

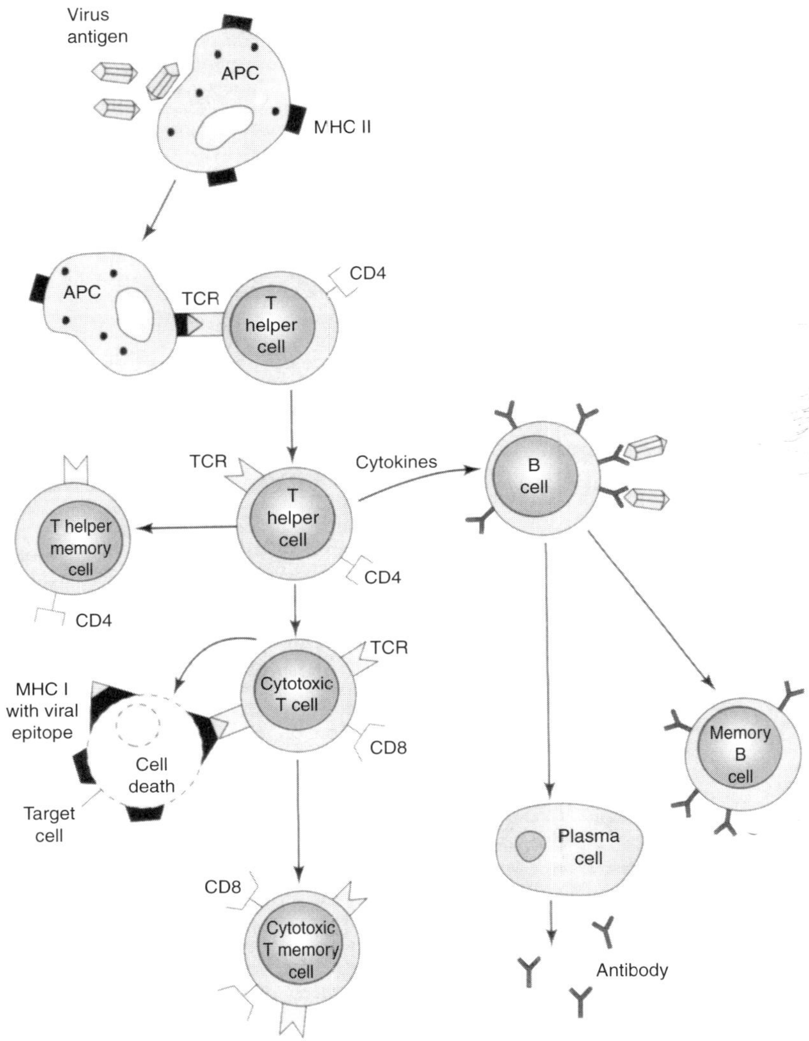

Figure 5.1 Immune cell function. MHC = major histocompatability complex, TCR = T-cell receptor. (From Porth, C.M., *Pathophysiology: Concepts of Altered Health States*, 5th ed., Lippincott, Philadelphia, 1998. With permission.)

Antibodies

- Also called *immunoglobulins.*
- Antibodies are globular proteins produced by activated B cells (plasma cells).
- Antibodies bind viruses, bacteria and toxins to inactivate them.

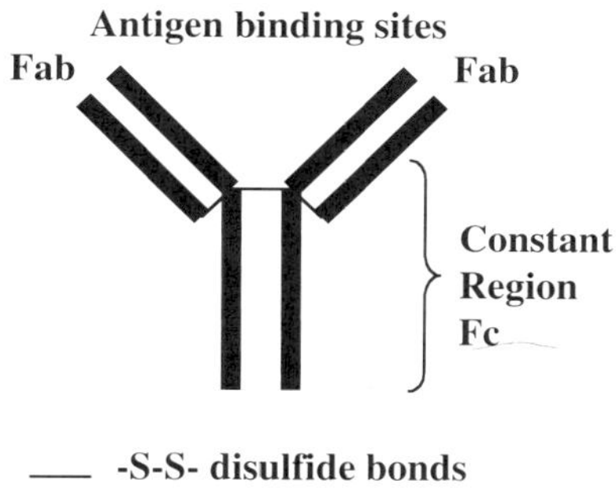

Figure 5.2 General antibody structure. Fab is the antigen-binding portion of the molecule, Fc is the "constant region."

Table 5.1 Antibody Characteristics

IgA	
	Predominant antibody in body secretions such as saliva, respiratory secretions and breast milk
	Protects mucous membranes
	Accounts for approximately 10 to 15% of all antibodies
IgG	
	Major class of antibody responsible for immune response
	Exhibits antiviral, antibacterial and antitoxin activities
	Accounts for approximately 80% of all antibodies
	Crosses the placenta and provides antibody protection to newborns
IgM	
	Largest antibody
	First antibody produced in an immune response
	Responsible for natural immunity such as ABO blood antigen reactions
	Accounts for approximately 10% of all antibodies
IgE	
	Binds to mast cells and is involved in allergic reactions
	Accounts for significantly less than 1% of all antibodies
IgD	
	Role in immune function is not clear but is required for maturation of B cells
	Accounts for less than 1% of all antibodies

- All antibodies share a basic common structure that is composed of two main regions: a *constant region* (Fc) and a *variable region* (Fab) (see Figure 5.2). The constant region is the same for all antibodies and performs mainly a structural role. The variable region differs between various antibodies and is the portion of the molecule that binds to the specific antigen.
- Five distinct classes of antibodies have been identified. Their functions are listed in Table 5.1.

Natural killer cells

- A nonspecific type of lymphocyte that destroys all foreign invaders by releasing cytotoxic chemicals and cytokines.
- Binds to any cells it identifies as "foreign" (e.g., that have altered or missing MHC I). Can also bind to and destroy antibody-coated target cells.

Cytokines

- Small proteins produced primarily by T cells and macrophages.
- The major classes of cytokines are listed in Table 5.2.

Complement proteins

- A system of more than 20 circulating plasma proteins that are activated in a cascade fashion.
- Complement proteins may be activated by IgM or IgG that is bound to a pathogen.

Functions of activated complement proteins include the following:

- Mast cell degranulation
- Bacterial cell lysis
- *Opsonization* (neutralization) of bacteria similar to antibodies

Table 5.2 Cytokine Actions

Interleukins (IL-1 to IL-17)
Inflammatory mediators
Stimulate proliferation and differentiation of T cells, B cells, macrophages and natural killer cells
"Chemotactic" factors for T cells and leukocytes
Interferons (α, β, γ)
Natural antiviral agents
Activate macrophages
Tumor necrosis factors (α and β)
Inflammatory mediators
Cytotoxic to tumor cells
Increase the activity of phagocytic cells
Transforming growth factor β
Produced by lymphocytes, macrophages and platelets
Chemotactic for macrophages
Stimulates the activity of fibroblasts for wound healing
Colony-stimulating factors
Produced by monocytes, fibroblasts and lymphocytes
Stimulate proliferation and growth of white blood cells and macrophages

The inflammatory reaction

Inflammation is the response of a tissue to injury. Although painful, the inflammatory reaction is essential for preventing infection of the injured area as well as for initiating the process of healing.

There are five "cardinal signs" of inflammation:

Rubor — The redness that occurs as a result of the increased blood flow to the inflamed area.
Tumor — Swelling of the inflamed tissue as a result of increased capillary permeability and fluid accumulation.
Calor — The increase in temperature (heat) that occurs in the inflamed area as a result of increased blood flow.
Dolor — Pain that occurs in the inflamed area as a result of stimulation of sensory neurons.
Functio laesa — Alteration or loss of function in the inflamed tissues.

The inflammatory response may be divided into main two stages: the *vascular response stage* and the *cellular response stage.*

1. Vascular response
   - Rapid vasoconstriction of blood vessels occurs in the injured area and is followed by rapid vasodilatation.
   - An increase in capillary permeability occurs in the injured area leading to swelling and edema. The fluids that enter the injured area are useful for diluting out any bacterial toxins or irritants present in the tissue.
2. Cellular response
   - Phagocytic *neutrophils* are the first white blood cells to arrive in the injured area. Leukocytes are attracted to the injured area by certain bacterial substances as well as by cellular debris and cytokines (*chemotaxis*).
   - As fluid leaves the capillaries, the viscosity of blood increases and leukocytes precipitate to the walls of the capillary. This process is called *margination*. Leukocytes undergo a change in shape and squeeze through the now more permeable capillaries into the tissues. The movement of leukocytes through the capillary wall is called *diapedesis*.
   - Other white blood cells such as *eosinophils* and *basophils* also arrive at the injured area and release substances such as *histamine* that enhance the inflammatory reaction. Histamine is a powerful vasodilator that increases capillary permeability. Monocytes will also enter the inflamed tissues where they mature into phagocytic macrophages.
   - Cytokines such as interleukin and tumor necrosis factor are released to enhance the inflammatory and immune response.

Prostaglandins are also released by many cells in the injured area and cause fever and vasodilation.

Hypersensitivity reactions

A hypersensitivity reaction is an enhanced and abnormal immune response. Hypersensitivity reactions may occur immediately or be delayed for one to several days. Hypersensitivity reactions are often referred to as *allergic* reactions with the offending substance referred to as the *allergen*. There are four types of hypersensitivity reactions.

1. Type I hypersensitivity reaction
   - Immediate hypersensitivity reactions that occur when an allergen binds to specific IgE antibodies that are attached to the surface of *mast cells*. These mast cells are found throughout many tissues and contain large amounts of the pro-inflammatory mediator *histamine* as well as other substances that enhance inflammation. Binding of the allergen to mast cell–bound IgE causes the rupture of the mast cells and the release of inflammatory mediators into the tissues. Circulating basophils also contain and release histamine that may be involved in this reaction.
   - Examples of conditions associated with type I hypersensitivity reactions include *atopic dermatitis*, food allergies and allergic rhinitis.
   - A very severe type I hypersensitivity reaction occurs with *anaphylaxis* (see below).

Anaphylaxis

Anaphylaxis is a life-threatening phenomenon that involves the very rapid and widespread release of histamine and other inflammatory mediators from IgE-coated mast cells.

Occurs in individuals who have been previously "sensitized" or exposed to a specific antigen.

Anaphylaxis is characterized by massive vasodilation caused by the release of inflammatory mediators. This widespread vasodilation can lead to marked hypotension and circulatory collapse.

Although inflammatory mediators such as histamine cause marked dilation of blood vessels, they are potent constrictors of bronchial smooth muscle that lead to marked narrowing of respiratory passages.

Other manifestations of anaphylaxis may include itching, flushing of the skin and gastrointestinal upset.

Question

How would you treat a patient who is experiencing anaphylaxis?

2. Type II hypersensitivity reaction
   - Tissue-specific reactions that involve the IgG or IgM antibodies attacking antigens on the surface of cells.
   - Binding of antibody to antigen leads to activation of the complement system and subsequent destruction of the cell through lysis.
   - Examples of type II hypersensitivity reactions include blood transfusion mismatch (ABO) reactions and *hemolytic disease of the newborn* that occurs when the mother's and infant's blood ABO or Rh proteins are incompatible.
3. Type III hypersensitivity reaction
   - Occur when circulating antigen–antibody complexes precipitate out of circulation and lodge in the walls of a blood vessel or in a tissue.
   - The immune complexes also lead to activation of the complement system and subsequent cellular destruction and damage.
   - The immune complexes themselves may become trapped in the glomerulus of the kidney, for example, where they trigger a localized inflammatory reaction that can lead to kidney damage.
   - Conditions in which type III hypersensitivity reactions occur include acute glomerulonephritis, *systemic lupus erythematosus* (an autoimmune condition in which antigen–antibody complexes form against collagen in the body) and *serum sickness* (a condition in which antibodies arise against foreign substances in the blood such as drugs, venoms and foreign blood antigens).
4. Type IV hypersensitivity reaction
   - A delayed hypersensitivity reaction that is mediated by T lymphocytes.
   - Cytotoxic ($CD4^+$) or helper ($CD8^+$) lymphocytes are activated by exposure to a foreign antigen. The activated lymphocytes in turn release inflammatory cytokines that lead to activation of other immune cells as well as the coagulation cascade. The end result is tissue inflammation and damage that may take hours or days to occur.
   - Examples of type IV hypersensitivity reaction occur with *autoimmune (Hashimoto's) thyroiditis* (see Chapter 18), delayed allergic reactions (poison ivy) and the reaction that occurs with the *tuberculin* skin test for tuberculosis.

chapter six

Acquired immune deficiency syndrome (AIDS)

Study objectives

- Describe the structure of HIV. What is HIV reverse transcriptase enzyme and why is it essential for HIV replication?
- List the three stages of HIV infection. Give the key characteristics for each.
- Define the term "opportunistic infection" and provide some examples of opportunistic infections in AIDS.
- Describe the mechanism by which the HIV virus infects a human cell.
- List ways in which the HIV virus is transmitted. What steps can be taken to prevent its transmission?
- Describe the various tests that are used to diagnose HIV infection.
- Define "viral load." What is its clinical utility?
- Describe the mechanism of action for each of the various antiretroviral drug groups. List common adverse effects for each of these drug classes.
- Discuss the problem of HIV drug resistance. Why might it occur and what can be done to combat it?

Introduction

Acquired immune deficiency syndrome (AIDS) was first identified in 1981 in a small group of gay men in the San Francisco area who presented with unusual opportunistic infections. In 1983, the human immunodeficiency virus (HIV) responsible for AIDS was first isolated. Today, according to the U.S. Centers for Disease Control[9] over 36 million people are living with HIV infection. It is estimated that nearly 22 million people have died since the epidemic began. In the year 2000 alone, it was estimated that 3 million people died from AIDS. Women are increasingly at risk for HIV infection; currently, 47% of adults infected worldwide with HIV are women. The developing world is especially hard hit by the HIV epidemic. It is estimated that 95% of people with HIV infection now live in developing countries.

HIV structure

The HIV virus is an RNA virus that belongs to a family of viruses called *retroviruses.* The flow of genetic information in these viruses is the reverse of that normally occurring in mammalian cells. For these retroviruses to replicate in infected host cells, they must utilize a special enzyme called *reverse transcriptase,* which allows the viral RNA genome to be first copied into a DNA/RNA hybrid and then into mRNA, which can be translated into new viral proteins by host cell *DNA* and *RNA polymerase*. Structurally, the HIV virus is composed of an inner protein *core* containing a double strand of identical (+/+ RNA) (see Figure 6.1). Also found within the protein core are specialized HIV enzymes such as reverse transcriptase and *proteases.* The inner protein core of HIV is surrounded by a second protein layer called the protein *shell.* The protein shell in turn is encased in a lipid bilayer called the lipid *envelope*. Protruding from the lipid envelope are numerous glycoprotein *spikes* or *peplomers* that serve as organs of attachment to host cell membranes. HIV peplomers are composed of two distinct glycoproteins, *gp41* and *gp120.* The gp41 serves to anchor the peplomer in the HIV lipid envelope; the gp120 serves as a specific binding site for the human cellular proteins called *CD4*$^+$ (CD is the acronym for cluster of differentiation). These CD4$^+$ proteins are found in greatest concentration on the surfaces of *helper T cells* (CD4$^+$ lymphocytes) and in lesser concentrations on *monocytes* and *macrophages.* When HIV encounters a CD4$^+$-bearing cell, the peplomer gp120 binds specifically to it at the CD4$^+$ site. This binding uncovers the gp41 on the HIV peplomer, which now embeds itself in the host cell membrane. Once *fusion* of the HIV has occurred with the host cell, the viral core (containing the HIV genome) is injected into the host cell. Within the host cell the viral core breaks down and the HIV genome is free to be replicated by the host cell machinery with the assistance of reverse transcriptase. New HIV viruses are formed as new viral proteins are translated by the host cell. These newly replicated viruses can leave the host cell by *budding* or exocytosis. The newly formed HIV viruses, however, are not fully "mature" or functional until they are enzymatically modified by HIV protease

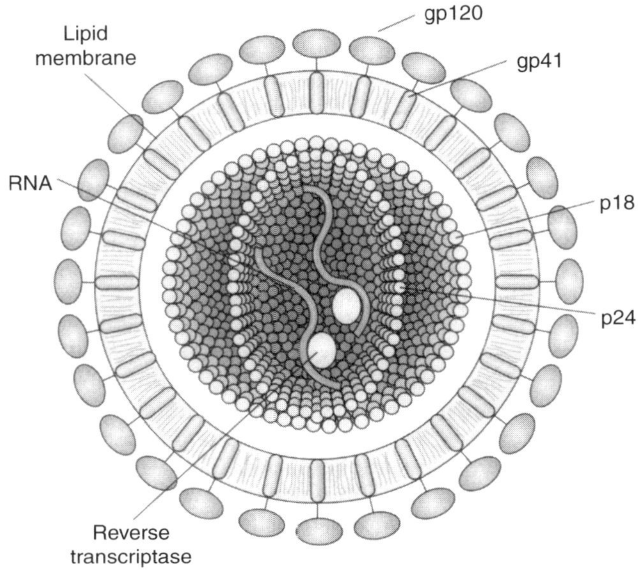

Figure 6.1 Structure of HIV. gp120 and gp40 are HIV glycoproteins involved in binding to host cells $CD4^+$. p18 and p24 are HIV structural proteins. (From Porth, C.M., *Pathophysiology: Concepts of Altered Health States*, 5th ed., Lippincott, Philadelphia, 1998. With permission.)

enzymes to the fully active and infectious state. A number of genetically different yet related HIV viruses have thus far been identified. Some of these variants appear to be particularly virulent since the progression of disease in patients infected with these strains is quite rapid. Other strains appear to be somewhat more "benign" as the disease progresses more slowly.

Stages in an HIV infection

Clinically, HIV infection presents in three distinct stages:

1. Acute illness stage
   - Generally occurs several weeks after infection with the virus.
   - Manifestations include acute-onset fever, headache, malaise, lymphadenopathy, sore throat and skin rash.
   - Symptoms usually subside within several weeks and the patient becomes asymptomatic.
   - During the acute illness phase there is a transient reduction in circulating $CD4^+$ and $CD8^+$ lymphocytes.
2. Asymptomatic stage
   - Following the acute illness stage, most patients go into a prolonged period where there are no symptoms of the infection. Patients

Table 6.1 Opportunistic Infections in AIDS

Pneumocystis pneumoniae — A parasite that can cause a severe pulmonary infection	Histoplasmosis — Generalized fungal infection
Candida — A fungus that can infect the oral cavity (oral "thrush")	Mycobacterium avium — Bacteria found in bird droppings, water and soil
Cryptococcal infection — A fungus that primarily infects the brain	Toxoplasmosis — A parasite that primarily infects the brain
Cryptosporidium — A gastrointestinal parasite that can cause severe diarrhea	Tuberculosis — Bacteria that primarily infects the lungs
Cytomegalovirus — Herpes virus that can infect the eye, intestine, esophagus, lungs or brain	

generally remain in relatively good health for 5 to 10 years. This asymptomatic period may be highly variable in duration.

- During this period there is slow but persistent destruction of immune cells, particularly $CD4^+$ lymphocytes. Toward the end of this period, circulating levels of $CD4^+$ lymphocytes decline significantly. Levels of $CD8^+$ lymphocytes may also show moderate decreases.

3. Symptomatic or AIDS stage
   - When circulating levels of $CD4^+$ lymphocytes fall below a critical level the infected individual becomes symptomatic.
   - A number of symptoms falling under the heading of *AIDS-related complex* (ARC) may occur. These symptoms include fever, night sweats, diarrhea and *opportunistic infections* (see Table 6.1). "Opportunistic" organisms are those that take advantage of the patient's weakened immune status to infect his or her system. Infections with many of these organisms are unique to AIDS or immunocompromised patients.
   - As levels of $CD4^+$ lymphocytes continue to fall, levels of HIV in the blood can increase markedly.
   - Malignant cancers may also appear as levels of $CD4^+$ lymphocytes continue to decline. The most common of these is *Kaposi's sarcoma*, a malignant neoplasm that can occur in skin, lymph nodes and viscera.
   - Neurologic manifestations are common in the late stages of HIV infection and can include *AIDS dementia complex* in which the patient suffers loss of memory, personality changes and loss of control over motor functions.

Epidemiology of HIV infection

The HIV virus is a blood-borne pathogen that is transmitted via contact with contaminated body fluids. Unprotected sexual intercourse (vaginal or anal) with an infected individual currently accounts for the vast majority of new HIV infections. The virus may also be spread through contaminated blood products (blood and blood factor transfusions) as well as through sharing of contaminated needles. Transmission of the HIV virus from infected mothers to their fetuses currently accounts for approximately 10% of all HIV infections. Because the HIV virus appears in breast milk, breast-feeding is not recommended in HIV-infected mothers. The HIV virus may also be detected in trace amounts in the saliva of infected individuals; however, there is no current evidence that the virus can be transmitted by casual contact.

Laboratory diagnosis of HIV

- Enzyme immunoassay (EIA) is used to detect HIV antibodies. A positive EIA must be confirmed by Western blot or immunofluorescence assay (IFA) to detect specific HIV proteins. HIV core protein p24 is the most abundant protein produced by HIV. Other HIV proteins such as p55, p40, gp120 and gp41 may also be part of the analysis.
- Although not used to diagnose HIV infection, measurement of $CD4^+$ lymphocyte levels and *viral load* (a measurement of HIV RNA levels in the blood) are often useful indexes of the disease progression as well as the effectiveness of antiretroviral therapy.[10]

Rationale for treatment of HIV

- Prevent viral replication in infected cells by inhibiting HIV reverse transcriptase or protease enzymes.
- Treat opportunistic infections when they arise and prophylactically.
- Provide nutritional, medical and emotional support for patients with a chronic illness.

Treatment of HIV

- The most effective way to limit the occurrence of HIV infection is through proper prevention (see Table 6.2).

Table 6.2 Prevention of HIV Infection

Practice safe sex
Condom use, abstinence
Prevent sharing of used needles among IV drug abusers
Implement effective screening of blood products in all countries
Increase voluntary HIV screening in high-risk individuals
Offer increased counseling on AIDS awareness and prevention

Table 6.3 HIV Drug Therapy

Nucleoside reverse transcriptase inhibitors
Examples: zidovudine (AZT), didanosine
Competitive inhibitors of HIV reverse transcriptase enzyme
Cause termination of growing viral DNA chain
These drugs require activation in the cytoplasm of the host cell to the active form
Common side effects include rash, nausea, diarrhea and peripheral neuropathy
Non-nucleoside reverse transcriptase inhibitors
Examples: nevirapine, efavirenz
Bind directly to HIV reverse transcriptase to inhibit it
Side effects include severe skin rashes, nausea, diarrhea and central nervous system effects
Protease inhibitors
Examples: saqiunavir, ritonavir
Inhibit HIV protease enzymes that are essential for enzymatic activation of newly replicated HIV viruses
Adverse effects include abnormal fat distribution ("buffalo hump"), hyperlipidemia, diarrhea, gastrointestinal disturbances and parasthesia

- Currently available antiretroviral drugs for the treatment of HIV fall into three categories: *nucleoside reverse transcriptase inhibitors*, *non-nucleoside reverse transcriptase inhibitors* and *protease inhibitors* (see Table 6.3).
- Considerable research is currently being conducted on developing an HIV vaccine that would protect individuals from HIV infections even after exposure to the virus.

HIV drug resistance

Emerging resistance of HIV to current drug therapies is a cause of great concern. The low fidelity of reverse transcriptase coupled with high rates of HIV replication and genetic recombination led to the emergence of numerous HIV variants, many of which are resistant to currently used antiretroviral drugs. The problem of HIV drug resistance may be partially offset by using several antiretroviral drugs in combination with one another. These HIV drug "cocktails" are highly effective in reducing detectable levels of HIV and have become a mainstay of antiretroviral therapy. Genotypic and phenotypic testing of HIV viruses for specific drug resistance is also gaining widespread acceptance as a possible tool for aiding clinicians in choosing the best drug to treat a particular strain of HIV[11] (see below).

HIV drug resistance testing

Genotypic resistance testing:

- More than 100 drug-resistant HIV mutants have thus far been identified along with many of the specific genetic mutations that confer the resistance.
- Genotypic testing looks for one or more of these specific resistant mutations in a particular HIV.
- Testing is generally rapid and relatively simple but can only detect a single or few mutations in any one virus and may not detect new mutations that have arisen.

Phenotypic resistance testing:

- Directly measures the ability of a particular HIV to grow in the presence of a specific drug or drugs.
- Can be a direct measure of drug susceptibility for a specific virus.
- Expensive and technically more difficult and time-consuming than genotypic testing.

chapter seven

Diseases of the vascular system

Study objectives

- Identify the components of a lipoprotein.
- Describe the role of each of the different lipoproteins in lipid transport.
- Describe the function of an apolipoprotein.
- List risk factors for development of atherosclerosis.
- Discuss the steps involved in formation of an atherosclerotic plaque.
- Compare and contrast the various genetic hyperlipidemias.
- What is an aneurysm? How may it occur? What is a dissecting aneurysm?
- List possible manifestations of an aneurysm. How can an aneurysm be treated?
- Compare and contrast Raynaud's disease and Raynaud's phenomenon.
- Discuss the etiology of varicose veins. How are they associated with chronic venous insufficiency?
- List factors that might contribute to formation of a venous thrombus.
- Discuss the role of anticoagulant and thrombolytic drug therapy in treatment of venous thrombus.

Introduction

Normal blood flow through arteries and veins requires an intact system of blood vessels and adequate perfusion pressure to drive the blood through these vessels. A number of disease processes can affect normal function of the arteries and/or veins. Disease-induced changes may impair blood flow through arteries and disrupt delivery of oxygen and nutrients to tissues while disease processes affecting veins will disrupt removal of waste products from tissues and the return of blood to the heart.

Arterial disease

Arteries deliver oxygenated blood to the tissues and organs. Arteries can vary in size from the large aorta that transports blood from the heart to medium-sized arteries that deliver blood to organs and finally down to small arteries and arterioles that feed blood through capillary beds. Arterial diseases include conditions such as *atherosclerosis, aneurysm, vasospastic conditions* and various *inflammatory disorders.*

Atherosclerosis

One of the most common diseases affecting arteries is *atherosclerosis.* It is caused by deposition of lipid *plaques* in the walls of arteries. While the formation of atherosclerotic lesions can affect any artery, the coronary arteries of the heart are the most commonly affected. Because dietary lipids and cholesterol are insoluble in the plasma, they are transported as part of complex called a *lipoprotein* (see Figure 7.1). A lipoprotein is composed of a hydrophobic core of cholesterol esters and a hydrophilic shell of phospholipids. A protein called an *apolipoprotein* constitutes the protein portion of the lipoprotein and is responsible for determining the metabolic fate of the lipoprotein as well as allowing it to bind to cell surface receptors for internalization. There are a number of distinct lipoproteins that are classified according to their density:

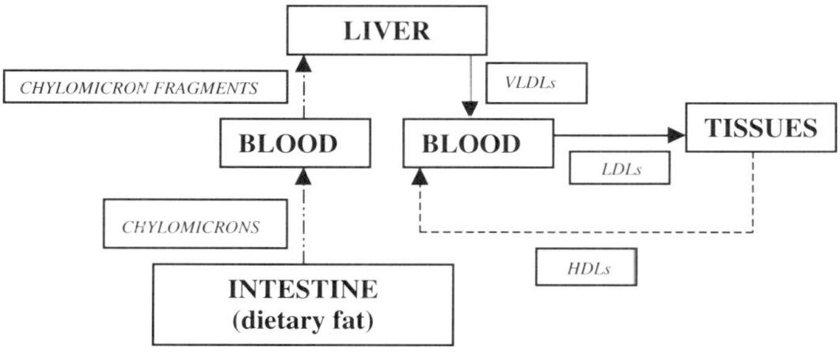

Figure 7.1 Lipoprotein transport and metabolism.

1. Chylomicrons
   - Lowest density
   - Synthesized in the gut wall
   - Mainly transport dietary triglycerides from the intestine into the blood
2. VLDL (very low-density lipoproteins)
   - Synthesized in the liver
   - Contains approximately 50% triglycerides with the remainder roughly equal amounts of phospholipids and cholesterol
   - May be converted to IDLs in the blood
3. IDL (intermediate-density lipoproteins)
   - Composed of approximately equal amounts of triglycerides, phospholipids and cholesterol
   - Precursor for LDLs
4. LDL (low-density lipoprotein)
   - Composed of approximately 50% cholesterol
   - Main carrier of cholesterol from liver to tissues
   - Internalized into cells bound to a specific cell-surface LDL receptor
   - "Bad cholesterol" due to its role in atherosclerosis
5. HDL (high-density lipoprotein)
   - Synthesized in the liver
   - Carries cholesterol from the tissues and plasma back to the blood
   - "Good cholesterol" because it removes cholesterol from the circulation; high circulating HDL levels associated with a reduced potential for atherosclerosis

When serum cholesterol and triglyceride levels are above normal the condition of *hyperlipidemia* is present. The association between elevated levels of serum lipids and atherosclerosis has been clearly demonstrated in a number of studies. The current general consensus in the medical community is that desirable serum cholesterol levels are those below 200 mg/dL. As serum cholesterol levels rise above this range, there is an exponential increase in the risk of atherosclerosis and especially disease of the coronary arteries. The cause of hyperlipidemia is often multifactorial and may include poor diet, sedentary lifestyle, or the use of certain drugs such as β-blockers and oral contraceptives (see Table 7.1). A number of genetic defects may lead to *hyperlipoproteinemia* (see Table 7.2). Some, such as *familial hypercholesterolemia,* are associated with a greatly increased risk for atherosclerosis and arterial disease. A number of key risk factors have also been identified that clearly increase an individual's risk for the development of atherosclerosis (see Table 7.3 and Figure 7.2).

Manifestations of atherosclerosis

- Tissue ischemia due to reduced blood flow.
- *Aneurysm* or hemorrhage due to weakening of blood vessel walls.
- Breaking-off of atherosclerotic plaques to form travelling *emboli.*

Table 7.1 Risk Factors for Atherosclerosis

Elevated serum levels of LDL
Low serum levels of HDL
Familial history of hyperlipidemia or atherosclerotic disease
Smoking
Hypertension
Age
> 45 years in males
> 55 years in females
Drugs — β-blockers, oral contraceptives, etc.

Table 7.2 Genetic Disorders of Lipid Metabolism

Five distinct forms of genetic hyperlipoproteinemia have been identified:
Type I — Familial hypertriglyceridemia
Autosomal recessive disorder (rare)
Greatly elevated levels of plasma triglycerides
Pancreatitis common but no evidence of increased atherosclerosis risk
Type II — Familial hypercholesterolemia
Autosomal dominant disorder
Caused by a genetic defect in the LDL receptor gene
Markedly increased levels of LDL cholesterol
Greatly increased risk of atherosclerosis
Type III — Broad beta disease
Mode of inheritance is unclear
Increased VLDL cholesterol and triglycerides
Greatly increased risk for atherosclerosis
Type IV — Endogenous hypertriglyceridemia
Genetically heterogeneous
Elevated VLDL and triglyceride levels
Moderately increased risk for atherosclerosis
Type V — Mixed hypertriglyceidemia
Genetically heterogeneous
Elevated VLDLs, chylomicrons, cholesterol, triglycerides
An increased risk of atherosclerosis has not been clearly demonstrated with this disorder

Table 7.3 Steps in the Development of Atherosclerosis (see Figure 7.2)

Formation of lipid plaques may be precipitated by endothelial injury (examples: hypertension, immune response, toxins in cigarette smoke, etc.).
Infiltration of cholesterol molecules into blood vessel walls.
Monocytes enter area of injury and release growth factors that stimulate smooth muscle and endothelial cell proliferation. Monocytes phagocytize lipoproteins and become lipid-filled "foam cells."
Platelets adhere to the endothelial lesion; fibroblasts infiltrate area and cause progressive *sclerosis* or hardening of tissue. *Calcification* of plaques may occur over time. Significant narrowing of the blood vessel lumen can occur over time.

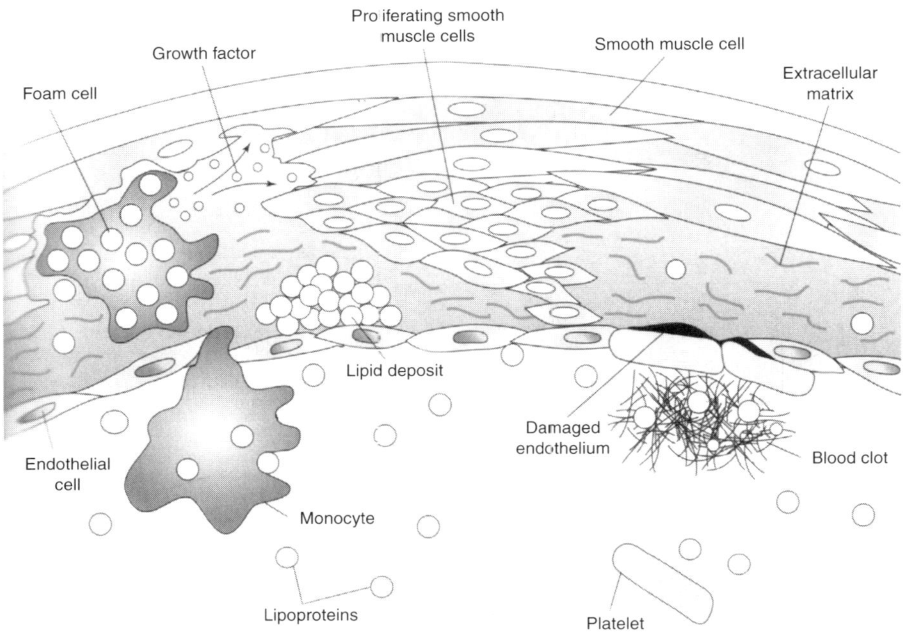

Figure 7.2 Initiation of atherosclerosis formation. (From Porth, C.M., *Pathophysiology: Concepts of Altered Health States*, 5th ed., Lippincott, Philadelphia, 1998. With permission.)

Aneurysm

An aneurysm is a localized, balloon-like swelling in the wall of an artery caused by weakening of the arterial wall. Aneurysm may occur in any artery, but the aorta is most susceptible to aneurysm due to the constantly high pressure on the walls of that vessel. Cerebral aneurysms may also occur. They are most frequently located in the *circle of Willis* of the cerebral circulation. A leading cause of aneurysm is atherosclerosis, as the formation of lipid plaques can erode arterial walls and compromise their integrity. Aneurysms may also be associated with hypertension, vascular infections and the normal aging process. Aneurysms that involve all three layers of the blood vessel wall are called *true aneurysms* to distinguish them from other types of arterial distention that may occur from external injury or trauma. A *dissecting aneurysm* is a very severe condition in which there is a tear in the inner layers of the blood vessel (tunica intima and tunica media) and as a result bleeding occurs in the space below the adventitia of the vessel (see Figure 7.3).

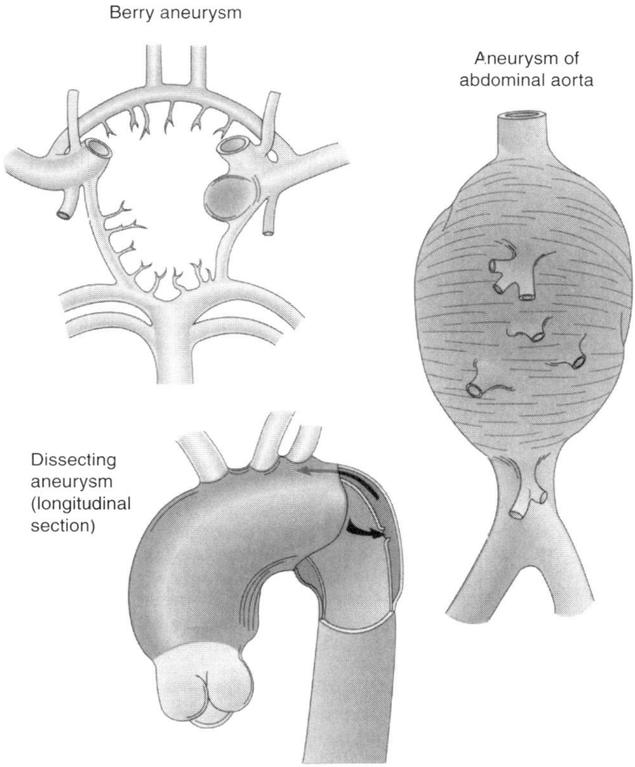

Figure 7.3 Aneurysm. (From Porth, C.M., *Pathophysiology: Concepts of Altered Health States*, 5th ed., Lippincott, Philadelphia, 1998. With permission.)

Clinical manifestations of aneurysm

- Depending upon size and location, aneurysms may be completely asymptomatic or may be associated with severe pain.
- Aneurysms in the *thoracic aorta* most commonly present with back or neck pain, cough, difficulty swallowing or compression of the trachea.
- Aneurysms in the abdominal aorta are often asymptomatic until they cause pain from compression on spinal nerves or abdominal organs.
- Aneurysms of the *cerebral arteries* often present with symptoms that are characteristic of increased intracranial pressure. Stroke can result if the abnormal blood vessel ruptures and bleeding occurs into the brain tissue.

Treatment of aneurysms

- Reduction of blood pressure and blood volume with appropriate drugs.
- Surgical grafting to strengthen arterial walls.
- Dissecting aneurysms are acutely life-threatening and require immediate surgical repair.

Vasospastic conditions

Two common vasospastic disorders are *Raynaud's disease* and *Raynaud's phenomenon*. These disorders are characterized by vasospasm of small cutaneous blood vessels in the fingers and toes. Raynaud's disease is a primary vasospastic disorder whose etiology is uncertain. It occurs most frequently in otherwise healthy young women and is often precipitated by strong emotions or exposure to cold. *Raynaud's phenomenon*, in contrast, is a vasospastic condition that occurs secondarily to other underlying diseases such as scleroderma, malignancy, or from blood vessel injury due to vibrations (jackhammers) or prolonged cold exposure (of butchers to low temperatures, frostbite). Localized vasospasm of arterial walls can acutely block blood flow to a particular region of tissue leading to numbness and discoloration. Severe or prolonged attacks of Raynaud's disease or syndrome may result in cyanosis, ulceration and gangrene of fingers or toes.

Treatment of Raynaud's disease involves avoidance of precipitating factors such as cold and strong emotions. Vasodilator drugs or calcium-channel blockers may be used to prevent vasoconstriction in Raynaud's phenomenon. In severe cases the sympathetic nerves that innervate the local vasculature may be surgically severed.

Arterial inflammation

Thromboangiitis obliterans (Buerger's disease) is an inflammatory disorder that can affect the aorta or peripheral arteries. It occurs most often in young men who are heavy cigarette smokers. The exact etiology of this disorder is uncertain but it manifests with inflammatory lesions of the arteries that may result in vasospasm, occlusion and thrombus formation. Treatment involves cessation of smoking and attempts to improve blood flow and reduce vasospasm through the use of vasodilator drugs.

Disease of the veins

Varicose veins

Varicose veins are veins that have become distended over time due to the pooling of blood in the lower extremities. This condition occurs most frequently in individuals who spend long periods of time standing (barbers, for example) or who have impaired return of blood from the lower extremities. Veins are thin-walled vessels that are easily distended by the chronic pooling of blood in the lower extremities. Chronic distention of veins can reduce effectiveness of one-way venous valves that are present in the lumen to prevent the back flow of blood and lead to a condition termed valvular incompetence (Figure 7.4). These venous valves work in conjunction with skeletal muscle pumps in the legs to move blood back to the heart from the extremities. The most common manifestations of varicose veins are aching and edema. Their appearance through the skin is also unsightly. Treatment often involves the use of support stockings to prevent venous pooling. Surgical interventions may also be used to improve appearance and reduce discomfort.

Chronic venous insufficiency

The presence of varicose veins and valvular incompetence can lead to a condition called *chronic venous insufficiency*. As a result of chronically impaired blood flow, congestion, edema and poor tissue nutrition, pathologic

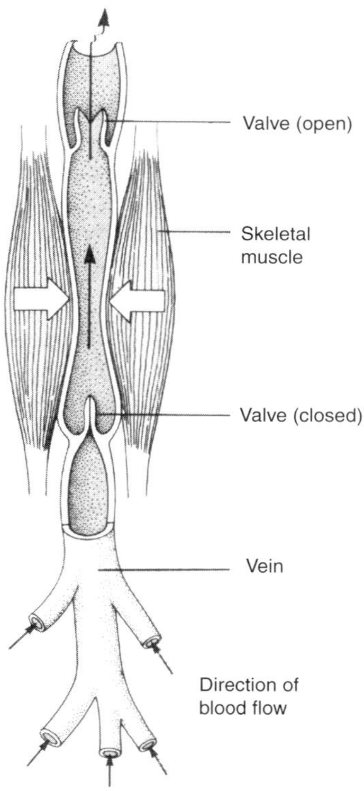

Figure 7.4 Venous valves. (From Marieb, E.N., *Human Anatomy and Physiology*, 3rd ed., Benjamin Cummings, Glenview, IL, 1995. Reprinted with permission of Pearson Education, Inc.)

changes may eventually occur in the lower extremities. Manifestations of chronic venous insufficiency may include skin atrophy, dermatitis, ulceration and tissue necrosis. Infection or trauma of the lower extremities that occurs in a patient with chronic venous insufficiency may have serious consequences because poor blood flow reduces delivery of immune cells and impairs wound healing. Treatment for chronic venous insufficiency involves interventions similar to those for varicose veins.

Venous thrombus

A *thrombus* is a blood clot that forms in the lumen of a blood vessel. A thrombus may form in an artery, but it is more common in veins due to the lower pressure and reduced blood flow found in the venous circulation. Factors that may contribute to the formation of a thrombus include the following:

1. Stasis of blood due to poor blood flow, immobility, heart failure, myocardial infarction and hypotension
2. Damage to blood vessels from trauma, surgery, IV drugs, catheters or immune response
3. Hypercoagulability of blood resulting from pregnancy, malignancies, coagulation disorders, dehydration or use of oral contraceptives

Thrombi may form in superficial vessels of the skin and extremities or in deep veins of circulation or tissues. Most superficial thrombi are benign and self-limiting, but *deep vein thrombus* (DVT) can be much more dangerous. Although a thrombus may present with pain, tenderness and swelling, it is estimated that nearly half of all deep vein thrombi are asymptomatic. As most deep vein thrombi occur in the lower extremities, painful compression or tenderness and swelling of the calf or thigh region might be used to diagnose a DVT in these areas. DVT are associated with significant mortality and morbidity and require intensive treatment.

Treatment and prevention of venous thrombus

- Prevent blood stasis in susceptible patients through ambulation, use of elastic stockings, exercise or elevation of legs
- Anticoagulation therapy (warfarin, heparin)
- Thrombolytic therapy to dissolve clots (streptokinase, TPA)
- Surgical removal of clots

Embolism

Unfortunately, for many patients with DVT the first manifestation of the thrombus is a *pulmonary embolism*. An *embolism* is a thrombus that breaks loose and travels through circulation. Common sites for lodging of emboli are the small pulmonary blood vessels of the lungs. Emboli that lodge in cerebral or coronary blood vessels may be rapidly fatal. A bolus of fat released by the breakage of long bones or an injection of air or foreign matter into the bloodstream through intravenous or intra-arterial lines can also act as an embolism. Ischemia and possible death of tissues may occur when blood flow is blocked by an embolus.

Anticoagulant and thrombolytic drug therapy

Anticoagulant drugs prevent the formation of blood clots by interfering with distinct steps in the blood-clotting cascade (see Chapter 3). Two of the most commonly used anticoagulants are *warfarin* (administered orally) and *heparin* (administered intravenously). Warfarin prevents the reduction of *vitamin K,* which is a cofactor necessary for activity of a key carboxylase in the clotting cascade. Heparin acts via an effect on *antithrombin III*. As a result of its mechanism of action, warfarin does not exert an anticoagulant effect *in vitro* (i.e., blood in test tube) whereas heparin does. Neither warfarin nor heparin has any action against clots that have already formed. Both drugs are bound to a significant extent to circulating plasma proteins that can alter their bioavailability. A main potential adverse effect of both warfarin and heparin is unwanted bleeding and hemorrhage. Drugs that inhibit microsomal metabolism, inhibit platelet aggregation or displace oral anticoagulants from plasma proteins can enhance the action of anticoagulants and increase the risk of unwanted bleeding.

Aspirin is a potent inhibitor of platelet aggregation through its inhibition of the enzyme *cyclo-oxygenase.* Inhibition of the cyclo-oxygenase enzyme reduces the formation of *thromboxane* A_2, a substance that stimulates platelet aggregation (see Chapter 3). Since platelet aggregation and activation appear to play a major role in thrombus formation, drugs like aspirin may be of significant therapeutic value in preventing their occurrence. A number of clinical trials have demonstrated the effectiveness of aspirin in preventing the tissue damage that accompanies blood vessel occlusion in arteriosclerosis and myocardial infarction.

Thrombolytic drugs are also known as *fibrinolytic* or clot-dissolving drugs. Unlike anticoagulants that prevent the formation of blood clots, thrombolytic drugs cannot prevent their formation. A number of thrombolytic drugs are now available for clinical use, including *streptokinase, anistreplase, alteplase* (tissue plasminogen activator) and *urokinase*. These agents promote the formation of *plasmin (*from *plasminogen),* an enzyme that degrades the *fibrin* proteins that make up the framework of a thrombus. The most common unwanted effects of these thrombolytic agents are unwanted bleeding and hemorrhage. Thrombolytic drugs have proved to be of clinical benefit in reducing mortality in patients experiencing myocardial infarction.

chapter eight

Alterations in blood pressure

Study objectives

- Distinguish primary hypertension from secondary hypertension.
- List the risk factors that may contribute to the development of essential hypertension.
- Discuss the major consequences of chronic hypertension. What target organs are most affected by hypertension?
- Discuss possible treatment options for essential hypertension.
- What are some possible causes of secondary hypertension? How might they be treated?
- Define malignant hypertension. Why is it so dangerous?

Introduction

Hypertension is defined as a consistent elevation of arterial pressure above the normal range expected for a particular age group. Nearly 25% of adults in the United States may have hypertension.[12] Approximately 90% of all hypertension cases are classified as *primary hypertension.* This form of hypertension is also called *essential* or *idiopathic* hypertension since its etiology is uncertain. Approximately 5 to 10% of patients are afflicted with *secondary hypertension* in which the cause of the elevated blood pressure is clearly defined.

Primary or essential hypertension

Although the cause of primary hypertension is still unknown, several theories involving chronic increases in fluid volume, enhanced sympathetic activity or abnormal salt and water excretion by the kidneys have been proposed to explain the mechanism of its occurrence. A number of key physiologic changes have also been observed in the kidneys of patients with essential hypertension that may contribute to the development of the disorder. These renal changes include increased resistance to renal blood flow, decreased renal blood flow with disease progression and inadequate excretion of fluid and electrolytes at normal blood pressures.

For a patient to be diagnosed as hypertensive, he or she must have had blood pressure measurements of 140 mmHg or above for systolic pressure and 90 mmHg or above for diastolic pressure at two successive measurements (see Tables 8.1 and 8.2).

A number of genetic, environmental and dietary factors are associated with an increased risk for the development of essential hypertension:

- Familial history of hypertension
- Increasing age

Table 8.1 Blood Pressure Measures

Systolic blood pressure = the pressure in the arteries when the ventricles are contracting
Diastolic blood pressure = the pressure in the arteries when the ventricles are relaxed
Mean arterial pressure = average blood pressure in the arteries, estimated as diastolic blood pressure + one third of the pulse pressure
Pulse pressure = systolic blood pressure – diastolic blood pressure

Table 8.2 Methods for Measuring Blood Pressure

Sphygmomanometer (blood pressure cuff) — indirect measure
Intra-arterial catheter — direct measure

- Race and gender: incidence of hypertension is significantly higher in black men
- High dietary salt intake
- Hyperinsulinemia
- Heavy alcohol consumption
- Obesity
- Cigarette smoking
- Low dietary intake of potassium, calcium and magnesium

Manifestations of essential hypertension

Although a small percentage of patients with essential hypertension may present with frequent headaches, most are asymptomatic. As a result, essential hypertension may go undetected and untreated for a number of years. Unless diagnosed early by blood pressure screening and treated appropriately, chronic essential hypertension can progressively damage tissue and organs, including:

1. *Blood vessels* — Prolonged high blood pressure in the arteries and arterioles will cause the walls of the blood vessels to thicken to compensate for the excess shear stress. The chronic increased shear forces that the blood vessel walls are exposed to also predispose them to atherosclerosis and aneurysm. As a result, untreated essential hypertension puts patients at a greater risk of coronary artery disease, cerebrovascular disease and renal vascular disease. The risk for atherosclerosis is exacerbated in hypertensive patients who have high serum cholesterol, are obese, have diabetes or who smoke.
2. *Heart* — Chronic elevation of arterial pressure means the heart must now pump blood out against a continually elevated afterload. As compensation for this increased afterload, left ventricular hypertrophy occurs. The hypertrophied ventricle will require increased blood, oxygen and nutrient supplies and will be at greater risk for arrhythmia. When the ventricular enlargement reaches a certain point, contractile function will no longer be supported and pump failure (congestive heart failure, CHF) will ensue.
3. *Kidneys* — Chronically elevated pressure can damage the renal vasculature and compromise renal blood flow, oxygen delivery and filtration. As a result, *renal insufficiency* can occur that may eventually progress to *renal failure*. Decreased renal blood flow can lead to activation of the renin–angiotensin system and contribute to a vicious cycle of increasing blood pressure and decreasing renal function. Hypertension-induced renal injury is exacerbated in patients with diabetes.
4. *Eyes* — Vision can suffer in a patient with chronic hypertension as a result of increased arteriolar pressure in the eyeball or from vascular sclerosis, both of which can damage the retina and eye as a whole.

Rationale for treatment of essential hypertension

Early detection of hypertension in a patient is essential to prevent organ and tissue damage. Comprehensive and frequent blood pressure screening is key. It has been shown that 31.6% of patients with hypertension do not realize they have it.[12] Once diagnosed, the treatment of essential hypertension is often multifaceted and will depend on the severity and responsiveness of the particular patient to various therapies. Management of the hypertensive patient should always include some modification of lifestyle and diet. In the mildly hypertensive patient, these lifestyle modifications alone might reduce blood pressure sufficiently such that pharmacologic interventions are not necessary. In moderate to severely hypertensive patients, pharmacologic interventions should be instituted promptly, in addition to lifestyle changes, to lower blood pressure and prevent the serious consequences of untreated hypertension. Patients who are diagnosed with hypertension at an early stage and who receive effective therapy for the condition will have a significantly lower morbidity and mortality than patients with uncontrolled hypertension. Regular blood pressure screenings are the key to early diagnosis.

Treatment

1. Lifestyle modifications
   - Weight loss
   - Exercise
   - Sodium-restricted diet
   - Cessation of smoking
   - Limiting alcohol intake
2. Pharmacologic
   a. Diuretics (*thiazides, furosemide*) — Lower blood pressure by reducing vascular volume. Thiazide diuretics inhibit sodium reabsorption in the distal convoluted tubules of the kidney, while loop diuretics such as furosemide inhibit sodium reabsorption in the thick ascending portion of the loop of Henle.
   b. β-Blockers (*selective* β_1 *and nonselective*) — Lower blood pressure by decreasing heart rate and cardiac output.
   c. Diuretics + β-blockers — This combination has been shown to reduce overall mortality in patients with hypertension.
   d. ACE (angiotensin-converting enzyme) inhibitors (*captopril, enalapril*) — Block the formation of *angiotensin II,* which is a powerful vasoconstrictor. Also reduces the formation of *aldosterone*, an adrenal hormone that stimulates salt and water retention.
   e. Calcium channel blockers (*nifedipine, diltiazem*) — Reduce blood pressure by relaxing vascular smooth muscle around blood vessels. Some calcium channel blockers may also reduce cardiac output.

f. Direct-acting vasodilators (α_1 *antagonists, hydralazine, diazoxide)* - Directly relax smooth muscle around peripheral blood vessels.
g. Central-acting agents (*methyldopa*) — Reduce blood pressure by decreasing sympathetic output from the brain.

Secondary hypertension

Secondary hypertension represents only a small fraction of all cases of hypertension. The underlying cause of secondary hypertension can usually be clearly elucidated and as a result can often be corrected or cured. One of the most common causes of secondary hypertension is *renal artery stenosis,* which is a narrowing of the renal arteries due to atherosclerosis. As a result of the reduced renal blood flow that accompanies the narrowed blood vessels, the kidney responds by activating the renin–angiotensin system that in turn leads to vasoconstriction and salt and water retention. Other causes of secondary hypertension can include *hyperaldosteronism* (excess aldosterone production) and *pheochromocytoma* (tumor of the adrenal medulla).

Secondary hypertension caused by renal artery stenosis may be effectively treated by ACE inhibitors or may be resolved with angioplasty or surgical intervention to reopen the occluded renal blood vessels.

Malignant hypertension

In a small percentage of patients with chronic essential hypertension, dramatic increases in blood pressure (greater than 120 to 130 mmHg diastolic pressure) may occur suddenly. These sudden increases in blood pressure are termed malignant hypertension and are especially dangerous because dramatic increases in pressure may damage the retina or kidneys and lead to cerebral edema and stroke. Malignant hypertension requires immediate medical treatment with powerful intravenous vasodilators such as *diazoxide* or *sodium nitroprusside.*

Hypotension

Hypotension is an abnormally low blood pressure. One common form of hypotension is *orthostatic hypotension* (also called *postural hypotension*) that occurs upon standing. The act of standing initiates a series of reflex responses in the body that are designed to prevent pooling of blood in the lower extremities and a decrease in blood pressure. These reflexes include vasoconstriction in the lower limbs and a reflex increase in heart rate. Some possible causes of orthostatic hypotension are listed in Table 8.3.

Table 8.3 Causes of Orthostatic Hypotension

Cause	Description
Aging	Associated with reduced baroreceptor responses, decreased cardiac output and reduced vascular responsiveness
Decreased blood or fluid volume	Caused by dehydration, diarrhea, diuretic use
Autonomic nervous defects	An inability to initiate vasoconstriction and increased heart rate reflexes
Prolonged bed rest	Associated with reduced plasma volume, decreased vascular tone
Drug-induced	Examples: antihypertensive drugs, calcium channel blockers, vasodilators
Idiopathic	Cause is not known

Manifestations

- Dizziness (*syncopy*)
- Decreased cardiac output
- Reduced brain blood flow
- Pooling of blood in the extremities
- Falls and injuries, particularly in elderly individuals

Treatment

- Maintain fluid volume.
- If patient is lying down, have the patient first sit for several minutes to allow blood pressure to equilibrate, then have patient stand slowly.
- Provide elastic support garments and stockings that may help prevent pooling of blood in the lower extremities.

chapter nine

Diseases of the heart

Study objectives

- Compare and contrast diseases of the pericardium. How can they affect cardiac function?
- What is myocarditis? What organisms may cause it? How does it differ from endocarditis?
- Distinguish the different types of cardiomyopathy in terms of their characteristics and hemodynamic consequences.
- What is rheumatic fever? How can it affect the heart?
- Compare and contrast the various types of valvular disorders in terms of causes, manifestations and hemodynamic effects.
- How can valvular disorders be treated pharmacologically and surgically?

Introduction

At the onset of the 21st century, cardiovascular disease continues to be a major source of mortality and morbidity in the United States. Nearly 50% of yearly deaths are attributed to diseases of the heart. Heart disease is a broad term that may include diseases of the *pericardium* (the sac surrounding the heart), *myocardium* (the heart muscle itself) or the *endocardium* lining the heart chambers. Various disease processes may also affect the coronary blood vessels that supply blood to the heart muscle or the heart valves that help regulate blood flow. Infectious agents, the immune system and congenital defects may also be important causative factors for a number of specific heart diseases.

Disorders of the pericardium

The pericardium is a sac composed of two thin layers of connective tissue that surrounds the heart. A thin layer of lubricating fluid called *serous* fluid separates the individual connective tissue layers. The inside of the pericardium surrounding the heart is filled with approximately 30 to 40 mL of clear fluid that prevents the contracting heart from rubbing against the walls of the pericardium.

Acute pericarditis

- May be idiopathic or caused by infection, ischemia, neoplasm, radiation, chemotherapy, immune activity

---

Idiopathic

A disease or condition, the cause of which is not known or which arises spontaneously.

Manifestations

- Chest pain
- *Pericardial friction rub* — Rubbing together of inflamed pericardial layers may be heard through a stethoscope
- Low-grade fever
- *Dyspnea* — Shallow breathing to avoid chest pain
- Electrocardiographic changes

Pericardial effusion

- Accumulation of fluid in the pericardial cavity
- May result from injury, inflammation, uremia, cancer, myocardial infarction, cardiac rupture, congestive heart failure or renal failure

Manifestations

- Not clinically significant until sufficient fluid accumulates to compress the myocardium.
- *Cardiac Tamponade* — Compression of the myocardium due to accumulation of fluid or blood in the pericardial sac (see Figure 9.1).
- Compression of the myocardium causes decreased cardiac output and venous return.
- *Pulsus Paradoxus* — A large fall in systolic blood pressure and stroke volume that occurs during inspiration. The presence of pulsus paradoxus may be determined by routine blood pressure measurement and is indicative of a possible cardiac tamponade.

Constrictive (chronic) carditis

- Chronic inflammation of the pericardium for months or years.
- May be idiopathic or can be caused by infection, uremia, radiation exposure, rheumatic fever, rheumatoid arthritis or chronic renal failure.
- Fibrous scar tissue and calcifications may develop over time in the pericardium.

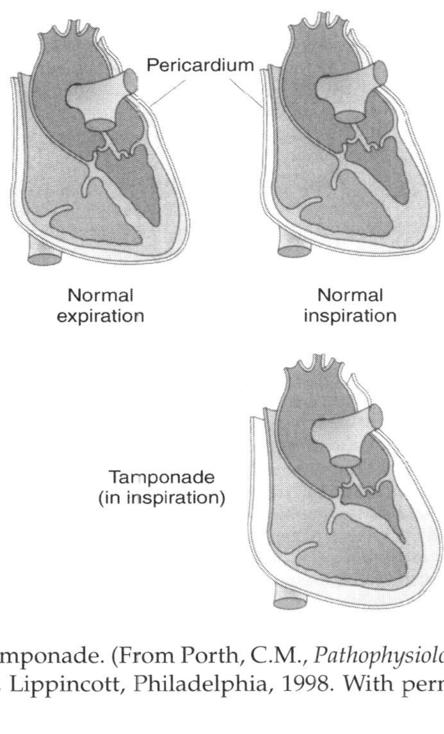

Figure 9.1 Cardiac tamponade. (From Porth, C.M., *Pathophysiology: Concepts of Altered Health States*, 5th ed., Lippincott, Philadelphia, 1998. With permission.)

- Scar tissue may eventually contract and restrict movement of the pericardium thus compressing the myocardium and interfering with cardiac filling and output.

Rationale for treatment of pericarditis

Treatment for pericarditis often involves relief of symptoms and if possible elimination of the causative agent(s). Analgesics may be used for relief of pain while anti-inflammatory drugs (aspirin, salicylates, nonsteroidal anti-inflammatory drugs, corticosteroids) can be employed to reduce inflammation of the pericardial tissues. Antibiotics may be initiated if bacterial infection is the cause of the inflammation. *Pericardiocentesis* or aspiration of accumulated fluid from the pericardial sac is often performed to relieve cardiac compression and reduce symptoms.

Diseases of the myocardium

Myocardial diseases are those that originate in the heart muscle.

Myocarditis

- Inflammation of the heart muscle without a myocardial infarction.
- May result from infection with viruses like *Coxsackie B* that replicate in heart muscle.
- May also occur with *rheumatic fever* (see below).

Manifestations

- May initially be asymptomatic but can present with flulike symptoms in the acute stages. Can progress to myocardial enlargement or congestive heart failure if chronic inflammation continues.

Cardiomyopathies

- Diseases of the heart muscle that may have an unknown etiology or that may be secondary to cardiovascular disease. The cardiomyopathies are classified into three distinct types: *dilated, hypertrophic* and *constrictive.*

Types of cardiomyopathy (see Figure 9.2)

1. Dilated cardiomyopathy
   - Characterized by gross enlargement of heart chambers that results in markedly reduced ventricular function.

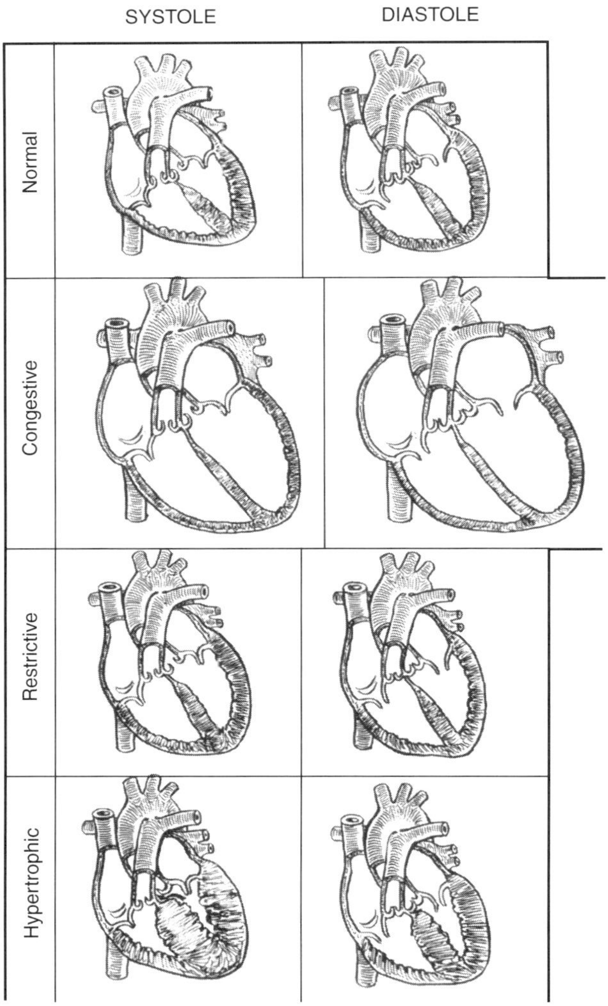

Figure 9.2 Cardiomyopathies: hypertrophic, restrictive, congestive or dilated, and normal. (From Price, S.A. and Wilson, L.M., *Pathophysiology: Clinical Concepts of Disease Processes*, 5th ed., Mosby, St. Louis, MO, 1997. With permission.)

- One half of all cases may be idiopathic. Remainder may be caused by chronic infection, chemotherapy, alcoholism or chronic myocarditis.
- Manifestations:

  Fatigue due to reduced cardiac output, dyspnea and pulmonary congestion.

  Arrhythmia may occur due to altered conduction in the dilated myocardium.

2. Hypertrophic cardiomyopathy
   - Massive enlargement (hypertrophy) of ventricles and septum that severely limits ventricular volume and cardiac output.
   - Although the cause of this disorder is unknown, there is an autosomal dominant gene that has been associated with this disorder.
   - Manifestations:
     Fatigue, angina.
     Arrhythmia, myocardial infarction and heart failure are all possible sequela.
3. Constrictive (restrictive) cardiomyopathy
   - A disorder characterized by excessive rigidity of ventricular walls.
   - Relatively uncommon disorder that may be caused by amyloid (glycoprotein) infiltration or glycogen storage diseases.
   - Manifestations:
     Excessive rigidity of ventricular walls limits ventricular filling and markedly diminishes cardiac output.
     Arrhythmia is common. May lead to congestive heart failure.

Rationale for treatment of cardiomyopathy

The congestive effects of cardiomyopathy on pulmonary and systemic circulation may be relieved somewhat by the use of diuretic drugs and with salt and water restriction. Bed rest can reduce workload on the heart, as can drugs that cause venous and arterial dilation. Digitalis glycosides may be used in dilated cardiomyopathy to enhance contractile function of the heart muscle (see Chapter 12). Anticoagulant drugs can also be employed to prevent blood clots from forming in pooled blood. In hypertrophic cardiomyopathy, β-blockers may be useful to slow heart rate and allow the ventricles a greater time for filling. Surgical removal of a portion of the hypertrophic ventricles may also be carried out to improve overall cardiac function.

Disorders of the endocardium and heart valves

The endocardium is the innermost lining of the heart walls. Disorders of the endocardium often spread to involve the heart valves that are continuous with the endocardium.

Infectious endocarditis

- Infection of the endocardium often caused by *Streptococcus* or *Staphylococcus* bacteria.
- Predisposing factors include previous damage to endocardium, intravenous drug use and systemic bacterial infections.

Manifestations

- Damage to myocardium
- Formation of emboli
- Destruction of heart valves

Treatment

- Antibiotic therapy
- Surgical repair of damaged tissue if necessary

Rheumatic heart disease

- Acute, recurrent or chronic inflammation of the heart that may affect the endocardium, myocardium and heart valves.
- May occur following throat infection with *group A β-hemolytic streptococci* bacteria, although the exact etiology is unclear.
- Primarily a disease of school-age children.

Manifestations

- The most serious manifestation is chronic disease of the heart valves that may markedly alter cardiac function and lead to heart failure a number of years later.

Disorders of the heart valves (see Table 9.1 and Figure 9.3)

Damage and dysfunction of the heart valves most commonly occurs as a result of inflammation or infection of the endocardium secondary to infective endocarditis or rheumatic fever. Damage may also occur through ischemia or direct trauma. Congenital defects or abnormalities of the heart valves may also be present in a newborn.

Two major types of changes are seen in heart valves: *stenosis* and *incompetence*.

Table 9.1 Heart Valves

Atrioventricular valves (two) — Ensure one-way blood flow between the atria and ventricles
1. Tricuspid valve: Three-flap valve located between right atrium and right ventricle
2. Mitral or bicuspid valve: Two-flap valve located between left atrium and left ventricle
Semilunar valves (two) — Lie at the openings of the aorta and pulmonary trunk Prevent the flow of blood back into the heart after contraction
1. Aortic semilunar valve: Lies at the opening between the left ventricle and aorta
2. Pulmonary semilunar valve: Lies at the opening between right ventricle and pulmonary trunk

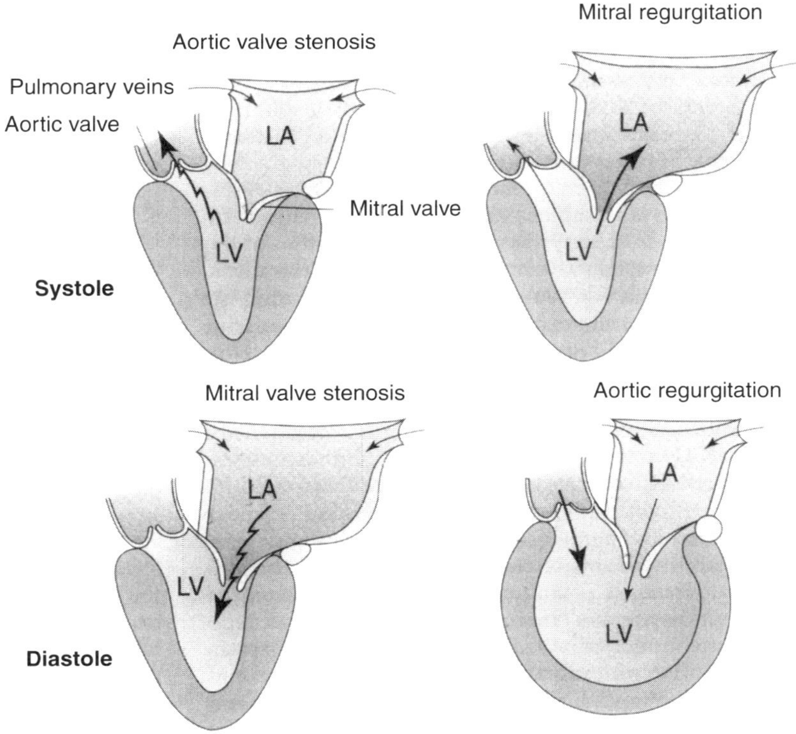

Figure 9.3 Heart valve defects. (From Porth, C.M., *Pathophysiology: Concepts of Altered Health States*, 5th ed., Lippincott, Philadelphia, 1998. With permission.)

1. Stenosis — Narrowing of the valve opening due to thickening of the valve walls. The result is a turbulent blood flow that leads to decreased efficiency of blood pumping and increased workload on the chamber that is pumping. *Aortic stenosis* affects the aortic semilunar valve and reduces blood flow from the left ventricle into the aorta. *Mitral stenosis* affects the mitral valve located between the atria and ventricles and reduces blood flow between those two chambers (Figure 9.3).
   Manifestations:
   - Hypertrophy of pumping chambers due to increased resistance to blood flow
   - Decreased cardiac output
   - Electrocardiographic changes, arrhythmia
   - Heart failure as a possible long-term consequence
2. Incompetent or regurgitant valves — Valves fail to shut completely and allow blood flow to continue even when closed. With *aortic regurgitation* the aortic semilunar valve fails to shut properly and

Table 9.2 Diagnosis of Valvular Disease

Auscultation — Murmur
Echocardiography
Electrocardiographic changes — Reflect chamber enlargement
Chest radiograph — Dilation of heart chambers or aorta
Hemodynamic change

some blood flows back into the left ventricle after contraction. *Mitral regurgitation* is characterized by a backflow of blood from the left ventricle into the left atrium during contraction.
Manifestations:

- Turbulent blood flow produces a prominent sound or "murmur" that can be heard with a stethoscope
- Hypertrophy and dilation of ventricles
- Eventual ventricular failure

Mitral valve prolapse

- A condition in which the upper edges of the mitral valves protrude into the atrium during contraction. The mitral valves are thickened and enlarged.
- The actual cause of the disorder is uncertain but it has a higher incidence in women than men, thus suggesting a familial basis.
- The disorder has also been associated with other diseases of connective tissue such as Marfan's syndrome.
- Although many cases of mitral valve prolapse are completely asymptomatic, some patients may experience fatigue, dizziness and atypical chest pain that is not associated with exercise (see Table 9.2).

Rationale for treatment of valvular disease

Pharmacotherapy of valvular disease often includes *diuretics* to reduce congestion and *anticoagulants* to prevent the formation of an embolism. *Vasodilators* can be of value in reducing afterload in mitral valve disease. *Antiarrhythmic* drugs may be employed if arrhythmias are present. Positive inotropic agents like *digitalis glycosides* can increase the force of contraction if heart failure occurs. *Antibiotics* may be given prophylactically to prevent endocarditis.

A number of techniques have evolved in recent years for surgically treating or correcting valvular defects. *Mitral valvotomy* involves opening of the mitral valve either surgically or with a balloon catheter. *Valvuloplasty* may be performed to surgically repair damaged valves or, if the disease is too advanced, affected valves may be completely replaced with graft valves (porcine, bovine or human) or with mechanical valves.

Congenital heart defects

Congenital defects of the heart are abnormalities that occur during fetal development. One of the most common congenital abnormalities of the heart is *patent ductus arteriosus.*

Patent ductus arteriosus

During fetal development the lungs are collapsed and blood is shunted around the lungs by a special blood vessel called the *ductus arteriosus* that connects the pulmonary artery with the aorta. When the lungs inflate at birth, blood flows through the pulmonary vessels and the ductus arteriosus occludes. In about 1 of every 5500 births this duct fails to close properly and remains patent. The presence of this duct allows for the backflow of aortic blood into the pulmonary artery. The turbulent blood flow can be detected on auscultation as a murmur. If not corrected, the continued pulmonary congestion places an excess workload on the heart that can result in heart failure years later. Surgical correction of patent ductus arteriosus is relatively simple and essentially involves ligation of the ductus arteriosus.

chapter ten

Myocardial ischemia

Study objectives

- Understand the relationship between myocardial ischemia and angina.
- Distinguish among classic angina, unstable angina, variant angina and silent ischemia.
- Provide a rationale for pharmacologic and nonpharmacologic therapy in angina and myocardial ischemia.
- Explain the mechanism of action for the nitrates, β-blockers, calcium channel antagonists, aspirin and heparin in treatment of angina.

Introduction

Myocardial ischemia occurs when the blood flow demands of the heart exceed the blood supplied by the coronary arteries. The leading cause of myocardial ischemia is *atherosclerosis* or blockage of coronary arteries due to the accumulation of lipid plaques and/or thrombus (see Chapter 7). Under conditions of rest, myocardial oxygen supply and delivery of nutrients through the coronary arteries should match the metabolic requirements of the heart. When the metabolic needs of the heart increase, the coronary blood flow must increase accordingly (see Figure 10.1). The myocardial oxygen balance figure lists several factors that will increase the oxygen and nutrient demand of the myocardium, as well as factors that can increase coronary blood flow.

With age and progressive occlusion of coronary arteries, smaller *collateral* vessels may begin to carry a greater proportion of blood and provide an alternate means of perfusion for an area of myocardium. These collateral blood vessels may run parallel to the larger coronary arteries and be connected to other small coronary vessels by vascular connections called *anastomoses*. Development of collateral circulation may reduce or delay the occurrence of symptoms from myocardial ischemia until the blockage is very progressed. The presence of extensively developed collateral circulation might also explain why many older individuals often survive serious heart attacks when younger individuals, who have not yet developed collateral circulation, often do not.

Manifestations of myocardial ischemia

Angina pectoris is the major symptom of myocardial ischemia. Angina pectoris most commonly presents as pain, pressure or a burning sensation in the area of the sternum.

There are three types of angina pectoris:

1. Classic or exertional angina
   - Pain is precipitated by increased workload on the heart. May be caused by exercise, emotions, stress and cold exposure.

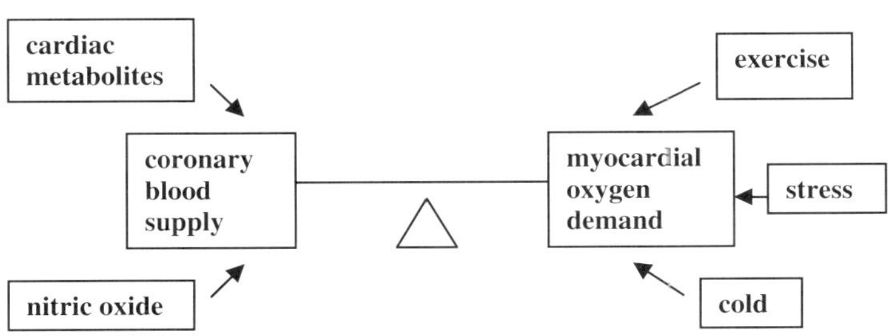

Figure 10.1 Myocardial oxygen balance.

- Symptoms may remain "stable" for a number of years or progress in severity.

2. Unstable angina
   - Angina that occurs at rest.
   - Also referred to as "pre-infarct" angina since it is usually associated with extensive blockage of coronary arteries. Coronary blood flow does not meet the needs of the heart even at rest.
   - Requires intensive treatment and evaluation.
3. Variant angina (*vasospastic angina, Prinzmetal's angina*)
   - Caused by vasospasm of the coronary arteries.
   - Usually associated with coronary artery disease but may result from excess sympathetic activity.
   - Frequently occurs at night, at rest or during minimal exercise.
   - May be precipitated by stress, cold exposure or smoking.

Silent ischemia is a particularly dangerous form of myocardial ischemia as there is a lack of clinical symptoms, i.e., ischemia without angina. Usually diagnosed by exercise stress testing or Holter monitoring (see Table 10.1).

Table 10.1 Diagnosis of Myocardial Ischemia

Electrocardiograph
Holter monitoring — 24 ambulatory electrocardiograph
Stress testing with electrocardiograph
Nuclear imaging
Cardiac catheterization

Rationale for treatment of myocardial ischemia

Treatment of myocardial ischemia and the resulting angina can involve two strategies:

1. Increase coronary blood flow by dilating coronary arteries
2. Reduce cardiac workload by reducing heart rate and/or force of contraction

Treatment of myocardial ischemia

The treatment regimen may include both nonpharmacologic and pharmacologic therapies.

Nonpharmacologic treatment

- Pacing of physical activity
- Avoidance of stress (emotional, physiologic, cold)
- Reduction of risk factors for ischemic heart disease (hyperlipidemia, obesity, hypertension, diabetes, smoking, etc.)

Pharmacologic treatment

Organic nitrates (Table 10.2)

- Dilate coronary arteries and increase myocardial blood flow.
- Dilate peripheral arteries and reduce *afterload.*
- Dilate peripheral veins and reduce *preload.*

β-Adrenergic blockers (Table 10.3)

- Block myocardial β-adrenergic receptors.
- Reduce heart rate and cardiac output (reduced myocardial workload and oxygen demand).

Question

Why would the use of β-adrenergic blockers be contraindicated in patients with heart block?

Calcium channel blockers (Table 10.4)

- Block calcium channels in vascular smooth muscle.
- Dilate coronary arteries and increase myocardial blood flow.
- Dilate peripheral arteries and reduce *afterload.*

Table 10.2 Organic Nitrates Examples

Amyl nitrate, nitroglycerine, isosorbide dinitrite
Route of administration — Inhalation, sublingual, oral, transdermal, intravenous
Long-acting forms such as isosorbide dinitrite used for prophylaxis of angina
Short-acting forms such as sublingual nitroglycerin may be used during angina attacks
Major adverse effects include headache, hypotension
Tolerance may develop rapidly

Table 10.3 β-Adrenergic Receptor Antagonists

Examples: Propranolol, atenolol
May be selective β_1 (atenolol), or nonspecific β_1 and β_2 blockers (propranolol)
Major adverse effects include bradycardia, reduced cardiac output, pacemaker depression and bronchoconstriction with nonspecific drugs
Many have rapid first-pass metabolism
Are also used for hypertension, arrhythmia and myocardial infarction, glaucoma

Table 10.4 Calcium-Channel Antagonists

Examples: Dihydropyridines (nifedipine), verapamil, diltiazem
Dihydropyridines have greater specificity for relaxing vascular smooth muscle
Verapmail and diltiazem have greater effects on cardiac pacemaker tissues
Major adverse effects include headache, hypotension, reflex tachycardia; risk of heart block of cardiac failure particularly with verapamil or diltiazem
Also used for hypertension and arrhythmia

Aspirin, heparin
- Prevent platelet aggregation.
- Use for prophylaxis of blood clots particularly in unstable angina.

Surgical treatment

Coronary angioplasty
- Uses a balloon catheter to open occluded blood vessels
- Usually performed under local anesthetic
- 5% mortality, high rate of vessel re-occlusion
- Use of metal "stents" in opened vessel reduces rate of occlusion

Coronary artery bypass graft
- Revascularization procedure in which a blood vessel is taken from elsewhere in the body and surgically sutured around a blocked coronary artery
- May involve multiple (one to five) blood vessels
- Re-occlusion of transplanted vessel is possible

Key terms

- Ischemia — Inadequate blood flow to a tissue or part of the body.
- Hypoxia — Deficiency of oxygen in tissues.
- Preload —The load on the heart at the end of diastole. Determined by end-diastolic volume.
- Afterload —The force that the contracting heart must generate to eject blood. Affected by peripheral vascular resistance and arterial pressure.

---

chapter eleven

Myocardial infarction

Study objectives

- Understand the etiology of myocardial infarction.
- Distinguish the types of myocardial infarction that might occur. How do they differ in terms of their myocardial involvement, location and severity?
- Understand the sequence of events that accompanies a myocardial infarction.
- List the major clinical and physiologic manifestations of myocardial infarction. Why does each occur?
- Discuss the role of cardiovascular compensatory mechanisms in myocardial infarction.
- Describe the complications that might arise from a myocardial infarction.
- Discuss the rationale for the various treatment aspects involved in myocardial infarction.

Introduction

Myocardial infarction or "heart attack" is an irreversible injury to and eventual death of myocardial tissue that results from ischemia and hypoxia. Myocardial infarction is the leading killer of both men and women in the United States. Most heart attacks are the direct result of occlusion of a coronary blood vessel by a lipid deposit. These lipid deposits may accumulate to the point where they completely block a coronary vessel or, more commonly, accumulated lipid plaques may break off from the vascular endothelium and act as a thrombus that blocks a coronary artery at a narrower point downstream. Prolonged vasospasm might also precipitate a myocardial infarction in certain individuals.

Coronary blood flow and myocardial infarction

The location of a myocardial infarction will be largely determined by which coronary blood vessel is occluded. The two main coronary arteries supplying the myocardium are the *left coronary artery* (which subdivides into the *left anterior descending* and *circumflex* branches) and the *right coronary artery.* The left anterior descending artery supplies blood to the bulk of the anterior left ventricular wall, while the left circumflex artery provides blood to the left atrium and the posterior and lateral walls of the left ventricle. The right coronary artery provides blood mainly to the right atria and right ventricles. Nearly 50% of all myocardial infarctions involve the left anterior descending artery that supplies blood to the main pumping mass of the left ventricle. The next most common site for myocardial infarction is the right coronary artery, followed by the left cicumflex. A myocardial infarction may be *transmural,* meaning it involves the full thickness of the ventricular wall, or *subendocardial,* in which the inner one third to one half of the ventricular wall is involved. Transmural infarcts tend to have a greater effect on cardiac function and pumping ability since a greater mass of ventricular muscle is involved.

Manifestations of myocardial infarction

1. Severe chest pain and discomfort — Pressing or crushing sensation often accompanied by nausea, vomiting, sweating and weakness due to hypotension. A significant percentage of myocardial infarctions are "silent" and have no symptoms.
2. Irreversible cellular injury — Generally occurs 20 to 30 minutes after the onset of complete ischemia.
3. Release of myocardial enzymes such as creatine phosphokinase (CPK) and lactate dehydrogenase (LDH) into circulation from myocardial damaged cells.
4. Electrocardiogram changes — Inversion of T wave, ST elevation, pronounced Q waves.

5. Inflammatory response from the injured myocardium — Leukocyte infiltration, increased white blood cell counts, fever.
6. Coagulative necrosis of the area of the myocardium affected by the infarction.
7. Repair of damaged areas occurs by replacement with scar tissue and not functional muscle tissue; therefore, some alteration in function is inevitable.

Complications of myocardial infarction

Depending on the extent of the area involved in a myocardial infarction, a number of complications might arise, including:

1. Rupture of weakened myocardial wall. Bleeding into pericardium may cause *cardiac tamponade* and further impair cardiac pumping function. This is most likely to occur with a transmural infarction. Rupture of the septum between the ventricles might also occur if the septal wall is involved in the infarction.
2. Formation of a thromboembolism from pooling of blood in the ventricles.
3. Pericarditis — Inflammation due to pericardial friction rub. Often occurs 1 to 2 days after the infarction.
4. Arrhythmia — Common as a result of hypoxia, acidosis and altered electrical conduction through damaged and necrotic areas of the myocardium. May be life-threatening and lead to fibrillation (see Chapter 13).
5. Reduced cardiac function — Typically presents with reduced myocardial contractility, reduced wall compliance, decreased stroke volume and increased left ventricular end diastolic volume.
6. Congestive heart failure may result if a large enough area of the myocardium has been damaged such that the heart no longer pumps effectively.
7. Cardiogenic shock — Marked hypotension that can result from extensive damage to the left ventricle. The resulting hypotension will trigger cardiovascular compensatory mechanisms that will further tax the damaged myocardium and exacerbate impaired function. Cardiogenic shock is associated with a mortality rate of 80% or greater.

Compensatory mechanisms for myocardial infarction

As a result of the hypotension and hemodynamic changes that accompany a myocardial infarction, the cardiovascular system initiates a number of reflex compensatory mechanisms designed to maintain cardiac output and adequate tissue perfusion:

Key terms

- Cardiac tamponade — Excessive pressure that develops from the accumulation of fluid in the pericardium.
- Pericarditis — Inflammation of the pericardium.
- Stroke volume — Volume of blood ejected from each ventricle per beat.
- End-diastolic volume — Volume of blood remaining in the ventricle at the end of systole (contraction).

---

1. Catecholamine release — Increases heart rate, force of contraction and peripheral resistance. Catecholamines can, however, be arrhythmogenic.
2. Sodium and water retention.
3. Activation of renin–angiotensin system leading to peripheral vasoconstriction.
4. Ventricular hypertrophy.

Unfortunately, these compensatory changes may increase oxygen demand and workload on the infarcted heart and worsen overall cardiac function.

Rationale for therapy

A main goal of intervention for myocardial infarction is to limit the size of the infarcted area and thus preserve cardiac function. Early recognition and intervention in a myocardial infarction have been shown to significantly improve the outcome and reduce mortality in afflicted patients. If employed in the early stages of myocardial infarction, antiplatelet-aggregating drugs such as aspirin and clot-dissolving agents such as streptokinase and tissue plasminogen activator may be very effective at improving myocardial blood flow and limiting damage to the heart muscle. Other drugs such as vasodilators, β-adrenergic blockers and ACE inhibitors can also improve blood flow and reduce workload on the injured myocardium and thus reduce the extent of myocardial damage. The development of potentially life-threatening arrhythmias is also common during myocardial infarction as a consequence of hypoxia, acidosis and enhanced autonomic activity and must be treated with appropriate antiarrhythmia drugs. Supportive therapies such as oxygen, sedatives and analgesics are also utilized.

Treatment for myocardial infarction (see Table 11.1)

1. Oxygen — Used to maintain blood oxygenation as well as tissue and cardiac O_2 levels.

2. Aspirin — If administered when myocardial infarction is detected, the antiplatelet properties of aspirin may reduce the overall size of the infarction.
3. Thrombolytic therapy — If employed in the first 1 to 4 hours following the onset of a myocardial infarction, these drugs may dissolve clots in coronary blood vessels and re-establish blood flow.
4. Vasodilator drugs — Intravenous *nitroglycerin* can increase blood flow to the myocardium and reduce myocardial work.
5. β-Blockers — Blunt the effect of catecholamine release on the myocardium, reduce heart rate and myocardial work.
6. Pain management — Sublingual nitroglycerin, morphine if necessary (see Table 11.2).
7. Antiarrhythmia drugs — To treat and prevent a number of potentially life-threatening arrhythmias that might arise following a myocardial infarction.
8. ACE inhibitors — Drugs that block activation of the renin–angiotensin system and thus reduce the negative effects of vasoconstriction and salt and water retention on the myocardium.

Table 11.1 Thrombolytic Agents Used Clinically

Streptokinase — Derived from β-hemolytic streptococcus bacteria; involved in the activation of plasmin
Anistreplase (APSAC) — Complex of human lys-plasminogen and streptokinase; Administered as a prodrug
Alteplase (TPA) — Recombinant tissue plasminogen activator
Urokinase — Endogenous human enzyme that converts plasminogen to active plasmin
Routes of administration - Intravenous. for all of the above
Major unwanted effects — Internal bleeding, gastrointestinal bleeding, stroke, allergic reactions

Table 11.2 Pain Management in Myocardial Infarction

Sublingual nitroglycerin — Potent vasodilator of coronary arteries, also dilates peripheral arteries and veins to reduce preload and afterload on the heart
Morphine sulfate — Powerful opioid analgesic that also provides a degree of sedation and vasodilatation; although the opioid analgesics have little effect on the myocardium, they are powerful respiratory depressants

Aspirin

- Inhibits the cyclo-oxygenase pathway for the synthesis of prostaglandins, prostacyclins and thromboxanes.
- Inhibits aggregation of platelets and is effective in reducing myocardial infarction, stroke and mortality in high-risk patients.

chapter twelve

Heart failure and shock

Study objectives

- Discuss the possible causes of heart failure.
- Distinguish left heart failure from right heart failure in terms of etiology and physiologic effects.
- Describe how right heart failure may result from left heart failure.
- Discuss the physiologic mechanisms that become active to compensate for heart failure.
- What are the clinical manifestations of heart failure? Why does each occur?
- Discuss the different approaches that might be used to treat heart failure.

Introduction

Heart failure is a condition in which the heart is no longer pumping blood effectively. Depending upon the cause, heart failure may be classified as low-output failure or high-output failure. Low-output failure is a reduced pumping efficiency of the heart that is caused by factors that impair cardiac function such as myocardial ischemia, myocardial infarction or cardiomyopathy. With high-output failure, the cardiac output is normal or elevated but still cannot meet the metabolic and oxygen need of the tissues. Common causes of high-output failure include hyperthyroidism (hypermetabolism) and anemia (reduced oxygen-carrying capacity), conditions in which even greatly elevated cardiac output cannot keep up with the increased metabolic requirements of the tissues.

Manifestations of heart failure

Classically, the manifestations of heart failure can be divided into those occurring as a result of *left heart failure* (left atrium and ventricle) and *right heart failure* (right atrium and ventricle).

Left heart failure

The left side of the heart is responsible for pumping oxygenated blood from the lungs out to the peripheral tissues of the body. The most common causes of left heart failure include myocardial infarction, cardiomyopathy and chronic hypertension. Left heart failure is also referred to as *congestive heart failure* due to the pulmonary congestion of blood that accompanies the condition (see Figure 12.1).

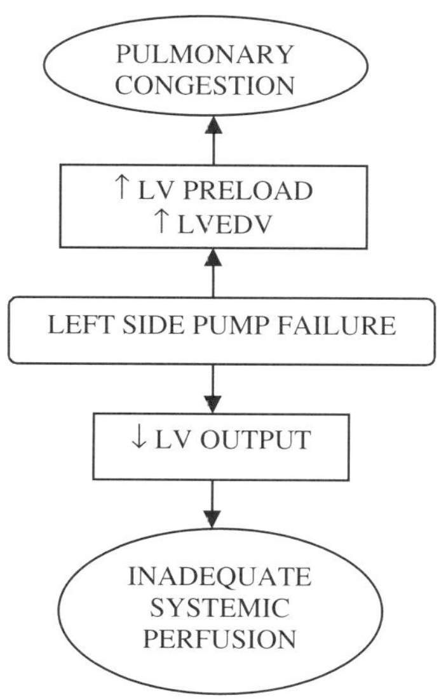

Figure 12.1 Consequences of left heart failure.

Manifestations of left heart failure include the following:

1. Decreased *stroke volume*, increased *left-ventricular end-diastolic volume* (LVEDV), increased *preload*
2. Congestion of blood in the pulmonary circulation leading to increased pulmonary pressure and pulmonary edema
3. Dyspnea, cough, frothy sputum; "rales" or crackling sounds that may be heard through a stethoscope as a result of fluid accumulation in the lungs
4. *Orthopnea,* the accumulation of fluids and dyspnea that are often worse at night or when the patient lies in the supine position because blood and fluids from the lower limbs may redistribute into the pulmonary circulation
5. Poor perfusion of systemic circulation that may lead to *cyanosis*
6. Generalized fatigue and muscle weakness

Key terms

- Stroke volume — The volume of blood pumped by one ventricle during one contraction.
- Preload — The degree to which the myocardium is stretched by venous return. Determined by LVEDV.
- LVEDV (left-ventricular end-diastolic volume) — The amount of blood that fills the left ventricle during relaxation.
- Ejection fraction — The fraction of the blood contained in the ventricle at the end of diastole that is expelled during its contraction (the stroke volume divided by end-diastolic volume).
- Afterload — The pressure the heart must overcome to pump blood out into the aorta.
- Orthopnea — Difficulty breathing when lying down.
- Cyanosis — Bluish discoloration of the skin and mucous membranes due to inadequate amounts of oxygen in the blood.

Right heart failure

Right heart failure often arises as a consequence of left heart failure. As a result of the increased pulmonary pressure that accompanies left heart failure, the resistance to blood flow now faced by the right ventricle is significantly increased as it pumps blood to the lungs. Over time, the increased workload on the right ventricle leads to dilation and eventual failure of the right heart (see Figure 12.2). Right heart failure may also result from chronic obstructive pulmonary disease, cystic fibrosis or adult respiratory distress syndrome (see Chapter 14).

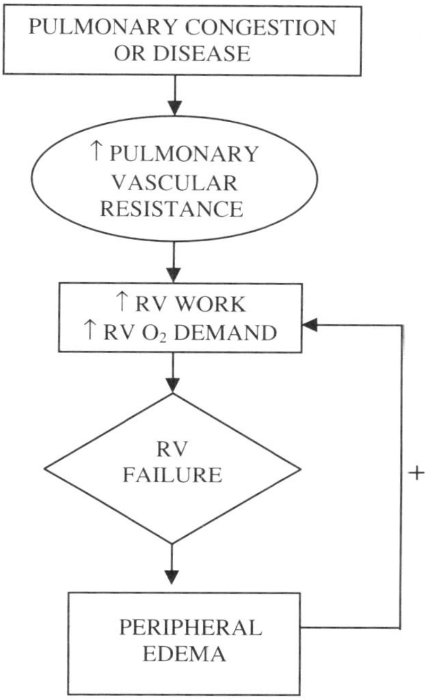

Figure 12.2 Consequences of right heart failure.

Manifestations of right heart failure include the following:

1. Increased right ventricular workload
2. Venous congestion and distention
3. Peripheral edema, ascites
4. Swelling of the liver with possible injury and eventual failure
5. Gastrointestinal symptoms

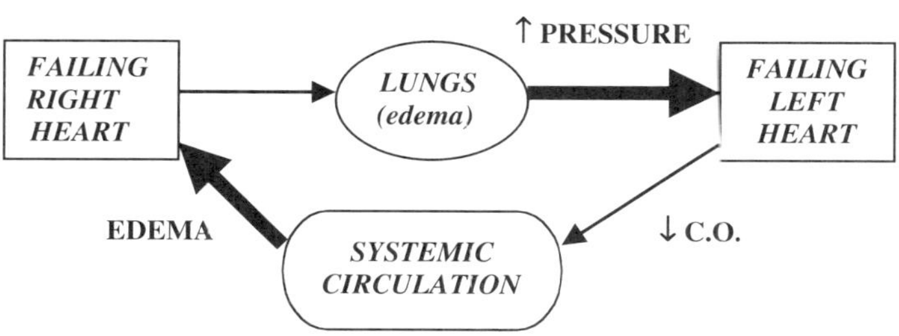

Figure 12.3 Circulation disturbances in heart failure.

Systolic failure vs. diastolic failure

Recently, the American Heart Association issued guidelines for treating heart failure based upon whether patients experience *systolic failure* or *diastolic failure*.[13] With systolic failure, there is a decreased ejection of blood from the heart during diastole. With diastolic failure, filling of the ventricles during diastole is impaired.

Systolic failure

- Decreased myocardial contractility
- Decreased ejection fraction
- Most commonly caused by conditions that impair contractility such as ischemic heart disease, myocardial infarction and cardiomyopathy
- Symptoms mainly those of reduced cardiac output

Diastolic failure

- Approximately 20 to 40% of patients with heart failure
- Preserved left ventricular systolic function but reduced ventricular filling that may be associated with impaired ventricular relaxation
- Associated with conditions such as restrictive and hypertrophic cardiomyopathy
- Symptoms primarily those of blood congestion and may include marked dyspnea and fatigue

Physiologic compensation for heart failure

The signs and symptoms of heart failure may not appear in the early stages as a result of a number of compensatory mechanisms that combine to maintain cardiac output. This early stage of heart failure is termed *compensated heart failure*. The compensatory responses are only effective in the short term and will eventually be unable to maintain cardiac output for a long period of time. *Decompensated heart failure* occurs when cardiac output is no longer adequately maintained and overt symptoms of heart failure appear. Compensatory mechanisms include the following:

1. Increased cardiac output — The normal heart responds to increases in preload or LVEDV by increasing stroke volume and cardiac output. The more the heart is stretched by filling, the greater its responsive strength of contraction (*Frank–Starling Principle*)[14] (see Figure 12.4). With heart failure there are chronic increases in preload that continually distend the ventricular muscle fibers. Over time, the compensatory Frank–Starling mechanism becomes ineffective because the cardiac muscle fibers stretch beyond the maximum limit for efficient

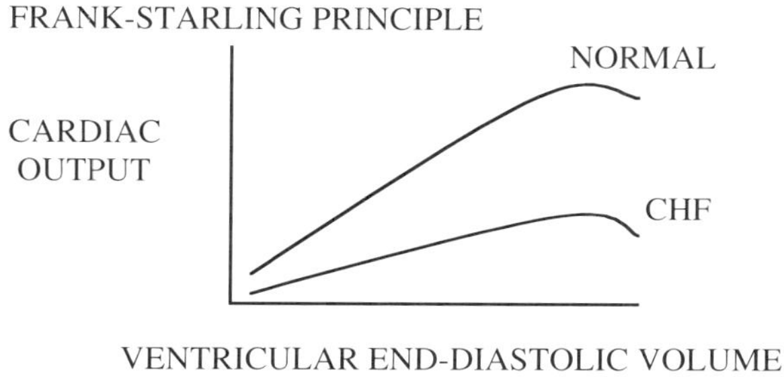

Figure 12.4 The Frank–Starling principle.

contraction. In addition, the oxygen requirements of the distended myocardium exceed oxygen delivery. At this point, further increases in preload are not matched by an increase in cardiac output.

2. Increased sympathetic activity — The decrease in cardiac output that accompanies heart failure will lead to decreases in blood flow and blood pressure that activate the sympathetic nervous system. The result of sympathetic activation is an increase in circulating levels of catecholamines that cause peripheral vasoconstriction as well as an increase in heart rate and force of cardiac contraction (positive chronotropic and positive inotropic effects). Unfortunately, the failing myocardium becomes dependent on circulating levels of catecholamines to help it maintain cardiac output. Over time, the failing myocardium becomes less responsive to the stimulatory effects of these catecholamines and function continues to deteriorate.
3. Activation of renin–angiotensin system (Figure 12.5) — As a result of decreased cardiac output, blood flow to the kidneys will be significantly reduced. The kidneys respond to this reduction in blood flow by releasing the enzyme *renin*. Renin ultimately leads to the production of *angiotensin II* in the plasma and the release of aldosterone from the adrenal gland. Angiotensin II is a powerful vasoconstrictor that increases systemic blood pressure while aldosterone acts on the kidney tubules to increase salt and water retention, a second factor that will increase systemic blood pressure. Other hormones that appear to be increasingly active during heart failure are *antidiuretic hormone* (ADH) from the pituitary gland and *atrial natriuretic factor* (ANF) that is released in response to atrial dilation. ANF may have a beneficial effect on CHF since it acts as a natural diuretic.
4. Ventricular hypertrophy — Faced with a chronic increase in workload, the myocardium responds by increasing its muscle mass. Although increased muscle mass can increase cardiac output in the short term, contractility eventually suffers as the metabolic demands of the hypertrophied myocardium continue to increase and the efficiency of contraction decreases.

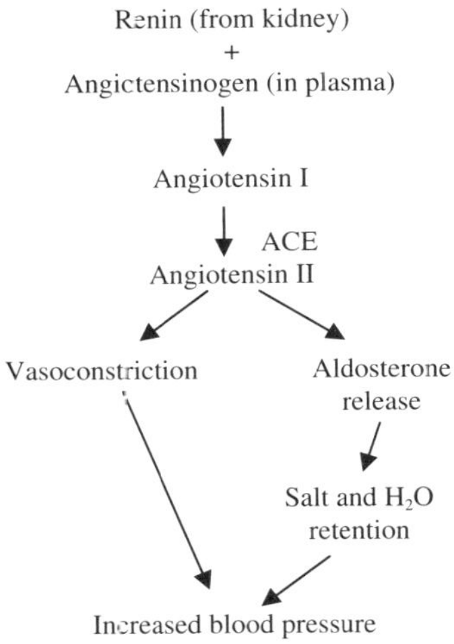

ACE = Angiotensin Converting Enzyme

Figure 12.5 Consequences of renin–angiotensin system activation in heart failure.

Diagnosis of heart failure

- Dyspnea with exertion, orthopnea, nocturnal dyspnea
- Rales, cough, hemoptysis
- Distention of jugular vein, liver enlargement, ascites
- Peripheral and pulmonary edema
- ECG, chest x-ray for cardiac hypertrophy
- Cardiac catheterization to assess hemodynamic function

Rationale for treatment of heart failure

Treatment for heart failure can be directed to reducing the workload on the failing heart and/or to enhancing cardiac contractility (see Tables 12.1 and 12.2). Treatment may include the following:

1. Restriction of physical activity to reduce cardiac workload
2. Reduction of preload through:
   - Salt and fluid restriction
   - Venous dilation with *vasodilator drugs*
   - The use of *diuretic drugs* to reduce fluid volume
3. Reduction of afterload through:
   - The use of arterial vasodilators
   - The inhibition of angiotensin II formation by *ACE inhibitor drugs*

Table 12.1 Drugs for Treatment of Heart Failure

Vasodilators
Organic nitrates — Dilate peripheral arteries and veins through relaxation of vascular smooth muscle; reduce preload and afterload on the heart
Arterial vasodilators (example: prazosin) — Cause dilation of peripheral arteries by blockade of α_1-adrenoreceptors; reduce afterload
Diuretics
Thiazide diuretics (example: hydrochlorothiazide) — Act on distal convoluted tubules of kidney to decrease active sodium reabsorption and increase fluid excretion; moderate potency
Loop diuretics (example: furosemide) — Powerful diuretics that inhibit the transport of sodium out of the ascending loop of Henle, leading to the loss of large volumes of sodium and fluids
β-Adrenergic receptor antagonists
Despite their potential for reducing cardiac output and force of contraction, numerous human studies have reported an improvement in symptoms, reduced hospitalization and decreased mortality in patients with heart failure receiving β-blocker therapy.[15] The mechanism of their beneficial effect is unclear but may be related to blunted catecholamine effects, reduced risk of arrhythmia, myocardial remodeling or improved cardiac energetics.
ACE inhibitors
Examples: Captopril, Enalapril
Block the formation of angiotensin II and aldosterone
Lead to a reduction in vascular resistance and reduced sodium/fluid retention
Positive inotropic agents
Cardiac glycosides (digoxin, digitalis) — Increase force of cardiac contraction by increasing levels of intracellular calcium in cardiac muscle cells
Other cardiotonic agents (dobutamine) — β_1-Adrenoreceptor agonist used for treatment of acute heart failure
Phosphodiesterase inhibitors (amrinone, milrinone) — Increases force of contraction through increased cAMP levels in cardiac cells

4. Blunting the effects of the catecholamines and adrenergic input with β-adrenergic receptor antagonists
5. Increasing contractility (positive inotropic agents):
   - Digitalis glycosides — digoxin
   - Inhibitors of heart-specific phosphodiesterases — amrinone, milrinone

With severe heart failure the last resort might be a heart transplant, although the current wait for transplant organs can be several years. Mechanical pumps called "left-ventricular assist devices" are currently available and can be used to take over a portion of the pumping function of the heart as a temporary measure. However, these mechanical assist devices are not designed as a long-term solution to heart failure. Considerable advances have been recently made in the development and implementation of self-contained mechanical hearts that are designed to be long-term replacements for the failing heart.

Table 12.2 Side Effects of Drugs Used to Treat Heart Failure

Vasodilators
Postural hypotension, headache, peripheral edema, reflex tachycardia possible with nitrates
Ace inhibitors
Hypotension, dry cough, possible renal failure in patients with renal artery stenosis
Diuretics
Thiazides: Glucose intolerance, hypokalemia
Loop diuretics: Hypokalemia, metabolic alkalosis
Cardiac glycosides
Narrow margin of therapeutic safety
Adverse effects include nausea, vomiting, arrhythmia
Marked effects on cardiac conduction that may be useful for rapid atrial arrhythmias
Increased toxicity with reduced plasma K^+
Mainly renal elimination, may have increased half-life in elderly individuals or patients with renal disease

Question

Why is the potential for digoxin toxicity significantly increased when loop diuretics are used?

Circulatory shock

Shock is a clinical condition of reduced blood flow to organs and tissues. Shock may be classified into three main categories based upon the cause of the shock. These categories of shock are *distributive shock, cardiogenic shock* and *hypovolemic shock.*

1. Distributive shock
   - Shock that occurs as a result of marked vasodilation and loss of vascular tone
   - Specific types of distributive shock as shown in Table 12.3
2. Cardiogenic shock
   - Shock that occurs when the heart is unable to maintain normal cardiac output
   - Possible causes of cardiogenic shock:
     Heart failure
     Myocardial infarction
     Cardiomyopathy
     Cardiac tamponade
     Pneumothorax

Table 12.3 Distributive Shock

Neurogenic shock
Caused by a defect in sympathetic input to the blood vessels
May be caused by brain injury, central nervous system depressant drugs or spinal cord injury
Septic shock
Occurs most frequently with systemic infection by bacteria
May be triggered by an immune response to bacterial endotoxins
Widespread vasodilation occurs in response to the release of inflammatory mediators (examples: histamine, cytokines) and bacterial toxins
Anaphylactic shock
Triggered by an allergic reaction to antigens such as drugs, food, insect venom, etc.
Develops suddenly and manifests with marked vasodilation, bronchospasm and hypotension
May be rapidly fatal

3. Hypovolemic shock
    - Shock that occurs from decreased blood volume
    - Possible causes of hypovolemic shock:
      Hemorrhage
      Excess fluid loss from diarrhea, vomiting
      Shifting of fluids from the vasculature to the interstitial spaces (*ascites*)

Physiologic responses to shock

Decreased blood pressure is detected by *baroreceptors* (pressure sensors) in the aortic arch and carotid arteries. Activated baroreceptors stimulate a centrally mediated increase in heart rate and cardiac output. The catecholamines epinephrine and norepinephrine are also released by the adrenal medulla to increase peripheral resistance, heart rate and cardiac output. Reduced renal blood flow will also lead to activation of the renin–angiotensin system with subsequent vasoconstriction and fluid retention. Up to a certain point, these compensatory mechanisms are able to maintain blood pressure and cardiac output; however, as shock progresses these compensatory mechanisms are no longer able to maintain adequate blood pressure and as a result tissue and organ perfusion will suffer.

Stages of shock

Shock occurs in three stages: mild (compensated), moderate (progressive) or severe (irreversible).

1. Mild or compensated shock
    - Blood volume loss less than 25% of total volume
    - Slight reductions in blood pressure

- Mild peripheral vasoconstriction
- Slight tachycardia (increase in heart rate), cool extremities
- Possible activation of thirst centers of the hypothalamus to increase fluid intake

2. Moderate or progressive shock
   - Blood volume loss on the order of 25 to 35% of total
   - Failure of compensatory mechanisms to adequately maintain cardiac output
   - Significant tachycardia and peripheral vasoconstriction
   - Tissues becoming hypoxic due to poor blood perfusion; possible *cyanosis* (bluish tinge)
   - Reduced urinary output (*oliguria*) to conserve fluids
   - Evidence of symptoms of poor central nervous system blood flow such as restlessness and impaired mental state
3. Severe or irreversible shock
   - Loss of blood volume that may approach 50%
   - Marked tachycardia
   - Rapidly falling blood pressure
   - Shallow, rapid breathing
   - Cessation of urine output (*anuria*)
   - Unconsciousness
   - Organ and tissue damage from hypoxia
   - Shock irreversible at this point even if blood volume is restored
   - Death from circulatory collapse

Complications of shock

- *Adult respiratory distress syndrome* (shock lung) — A potentially fatal respiratory failure that accompanies severe shock. The exact cause is uncertain but the condition may involve ischemic injury to lung tissues.
- Acute renal failure due to reduced renal perfusion.
- *Disseminated intravascular coagulation* — Formation of multiple small blood clots that may be related to sluggish blood flow or abnormal clotting activity.
- Multiple organ failure, cerebral hypoxia, death.

Rationale for therapy

The underlying cause of the shock must be corrected if possible. Plasma volume must also be restored through the administration of fluids, plasma or blood. Drugs that affect vascular tone or cardiac output may also be of value.

Treatment of shock

- Administration of intravenous fluids; possible incorporation of plasma expanders such as dextran and albumin
- Maintenance of airways, mechanical ventilation
- Administration of packed red cells for hemorrhagic shock
- *Vasoactive drugs* such as *dopamine* that causes vasoconstriction to skin and muscle while increasing blood flow to vital organs
- Vasodilator drugs such as *nitroprusside* that may be useful for relieving workload on the heart in cases of cardiogenic shock

chapter thirteen

Abnormalities of cardiac conduction

Study objectives

- Describe how cardiac pacemaker cells differ from ordinary cardiac muscle cells.
- Describe the conduction and pacemaker systems of the heart.
- What does each segment of the electrocardiogram represent?
- Discuss the two mechanisms by which an arrhythmia can arise.
- Describe the key features of the various types of atrial and ventricular arrhythmias.
- Define heart block and distinguish between first-, second- and third-degree heart block.
- Discuss the rationale and various treatment options for cardiac arrhythmias.

Introduction

A cardiac arrhythmia or dysrhythmia is any disturbance that occurs to normal heart rhythm. Cardiac arrhythmias can vary in severity from an occasional missed beat to serious abnormalities of rate and rhythm that severely impair the pumping ability of the heart and can be rapidly life-threatening. Abnormal cardiac rhythms can arise in tissues of the atria or ventricles and often involve derangements to the normal cardiac conduction pathways described below (see Figure 13.1).

Cardiac conduction system

Heart muscle is a unique tissue in that it has the capability of both *generating* and *conducting* electrical impulses. Specialized cells of the heart called *pacemaker cells* have the property of *automaticity,* which means they can spontaneously depolarize to generate an action potential. The primary components of the cardiac conduction system include the following:

1. Sinoatrial (SA) node
   - Located in the wall of the right atrium
   - Primary pacemaker of the heart that sets normal rate and rhythm
   - Depolarizes spontaneously 60 to 100 times per minute to set the resting heart rate
   - Transmits depolarization impulses to AV node via *conduction bundles*

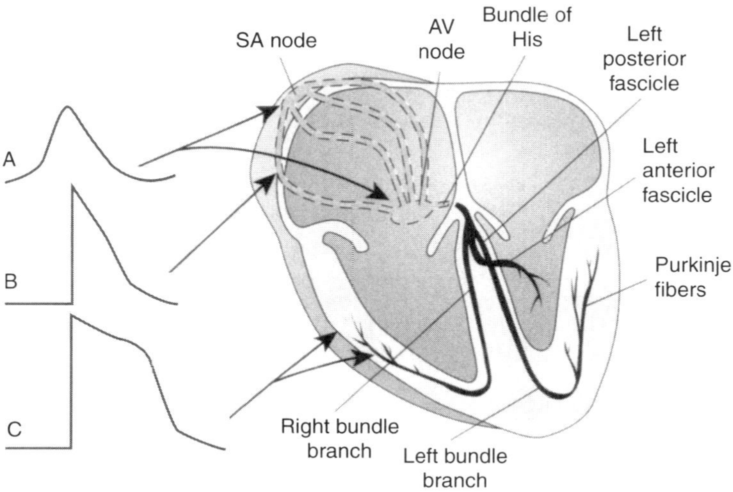

Figure 13.1 Cardiac conduction system. (From Porth, C.M., *Pathophysiology: Concepts of Altered Health States,* 5th ed., Lippincott, Philadelphia, 1998. With permission.)

2. Atrioventricular (AV) node
   - Located in the posterior wall of the septum
   - Receives impulses from the SA node and transmits them via the *bundle of His* through the ventricular septum
   - May take over as primary pacemaker if the SA node is defective, but at a slower rate of depolarization
3. Left and right bundle branch
   - Conducts electrical impulses from the AV node and bundle of His down the ventricular septum to the *apex* of the ventricles
4. Purkinje fibers
   - Highly branched fibers that carry electrical impulses up through the muscle mass of the ventricles
   - May act as a tertiary pacemaker in the event of SA and AV node failure but have a very low rate of depolarization that yields a very low cardiac output if pacing the heart

Cardiac action potentials

The cell membranes of cardiac muscle cells are *polarized* at rest (+ outside, – inside) and impermeable to sodium, potassium and calcium ions. When an electrical impulse is generated by pacemaker cells, a depolarization of cardiac muscle cells occurs that is accompanied by the opening of sodium, potassium and calcium channels in the cell membrane (see Figure 13.2).

Phases of cardiac muscle cell action potential

Phase 0 — Opening of Na^+ channels, rapid depolarization of cell membrane
Phase 1 — Inactivation of Na^+ channels, some small influx of Cl^- occurs
Phase 2 — *Plateau phase*, some K^+ efflux, Ca^{2+} enters for actual muscle contraction
Phase 3 — Rapid outward movement of K^+ that reestablishes resting membrane potential, but Na^+ and K^+ ions on the wrong side of the membrane
Phase 4 — Active Na^+–K^+ pump, which switches location of ions and restores normal resting membrane potential

Phases of action potential for cardiac pacemaker cells

Cardiac pacemaker cells (SA node) depolarize spontaneously due to a "leakiness" of their cell membranes that allows Na^+ ions to flow slowly inward.

Phase 4 — Slow inward leak of Na^+ causes spontaneous depolarization to threshold potential.

Note: The *slope* of Phase 4 (i.e., rate of firing of pacemakers) may be influenced directly through the actions of such substances as catecholamines, acetylcholine and various drugs.

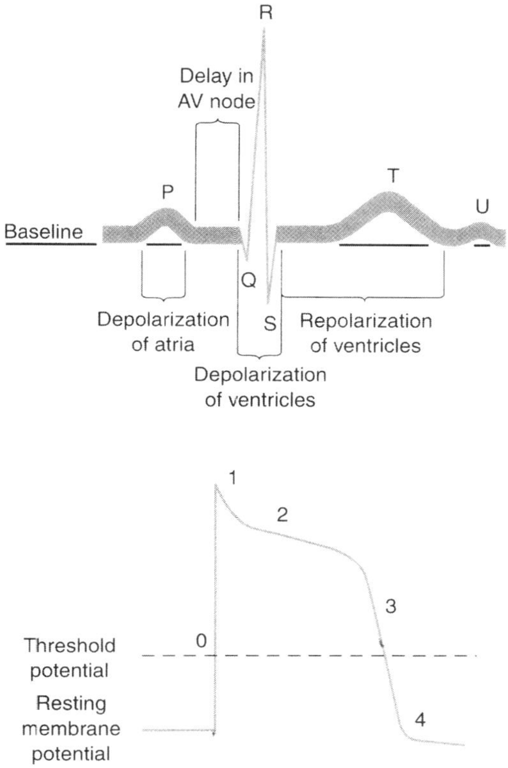

Figure 13.2 Normal electrocardiogram (top). Cardiac muscle cell action potential (bottom). (From Porth, C.M., *Pathophysiology: Concepts of Altered Health States*, 5th ed., Lippincott, Philadelphia, 1998. With permission.)

Key terms

- Threshold potential — The minimum depolarization required to initiate an action potential.
- Conduction velocity — Rate at which electrical impulses are carried through the myocardium; directly affected by the speed of the action potential in various cells.
- Absolute refractory period — A period of time immediately following an action potential during which a second action potential cannot be triggered by a stimulus of any size.
- Relative refractory period — A period immediately following an action potential during which a greater-than-normal stimuli can start another action potential.

Phase 0 — Continued influx of Na^+ and rapid influx of Ca^{2+}. Depolarization of pacemaker cells is largely dependent upon influx of calcium unlike cardiac muscle cells.
Phase 3 — Efflux of K^+ from cells.

Electrocardiography

The *electrocardiogram* (ECG) is used to measure electrical activity of the heart. Electrocardiography is performed by placing recording electrodes on the surfaces of the left and right forearm and left ankle to measure the electrical activity of the heart that is conducted to the surface of the skin (see Figure 13.2).

Components of a normal ECG

1. P Wave — Depolarization of the atria
2. P-Q Interval — Conduction through AV node, bundle of His, bundle branches and Purkinje fibers
3. QRS Complex — Depolarization of ventricles
4. T Wave — Repolarization of ventricles; note that the repolarization of the atria is lost in the QRS complex

Factors that may contribute to the development of a cardiac arrhythmia

A number of different physiologic factors and conditions may alter normal cardiac pacemaker or muscle cell physiology and lead to the development of a cardiac arrhythmia:

- Ischemia
- Myocardial infarction
- Electrolyte imbalance
- Altered cellular pH
- Administration of certain drugs
- Congenital defects in the heart

Mechanisms of cardiac arrhythmia

There are two clearly defined cellular mechanisms by which a cardiac arrhythmia might arise. These mechanisms involve *ectopic pacemakers* or *reentry impulses*. Ectopic pacemakers or reentry impulses may arise in the cardiac conduction pathways or in muscle cells of the atria or ventricles.

Ectopic pacemakers

The term *ectopic* refers to the occurrence of displaced or abnormal pacemakers in the heart. Under certain conditions, activity of the SA node may be suppressed and other regions of the myocardium that are capable of automaticity take over as the primary pacemaker, assuming control over the rate and rhythm of the heart. Also, as a result of ischemia, hypoxia and altered pH, cardiac cells that might not normally function as pacemakers now become excitable and can act as a second or "ectopic" pacemaker. Firing of these ectopic pacemakers can lead to premature cardiac depolarizations that do not follow the normal conduction system of the heart and that are in conflict with those arising from the SA node.

Reentry impulses

In a normally functioning myocardium, electrical impulses originating in the SA node follow an orderly progression through the conduction system of the atria and ventricles. These depolarization impulses cannot reenter cardiac tissue that has already been depolarized behind it and terminate after the ventricles are depolarized. In an abnormal myocardium, conditions might exist in which there is an area of slowed electrical conduction coupled with a one-way conduction block. Because of the slow rate of depolarization and one-way conduction block, it may be possible for depolarization impulses to travel back upward through the area of one-way conduction block and to "reenter" into higher areas of the myocardium, which, as a result of the slowed conduction, may have had time to repolarize. Thus, a single wave of depolarization may cause more than one beat. If the timing of reentry is right and the impulse impinges on the area of myocardium it is entering after the refractory period has occurred, a self-perpetuating "circuitous" type of electrical depolarization might occur (see Figure 13.3).

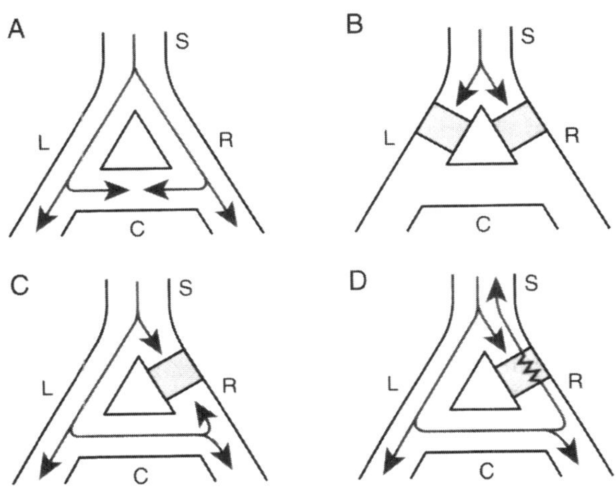

Figure 13.3 (A) Normal conduction; (B) two-way conduction block; (C) one-way conduction block; (D) reentry current. (From Porth, C.M., *Pathophysiology: Concepts of Altered Health States*, 5th ed., Lippincott, Philadelphia, 1998. With permission.)

Types of arrhythmia

Sinus node arrhythmia

- *Sinus bradycardia* — Excessively slow heart rate (<60 beats per minute, bpm)
- *Sinus tachycardia* — Excessively fast heart rate (>100 bpm)
- *Sinus arrest* — Failure of SA node to discharge, secondary pacemakers may take over (i.e., AV node)

Atrial arrhythmia (Figure 13.4)

- Premature atrial contractions
  Contraction of the heart before the normal contraction
  Most occur from ectopic impulses
  Also called *premature beats* or *extrasystole*
- Atrial paroxysmal tachycardia
  Sudden increase in atrial contraction rate to approximately 150 bpm
- Atrial flutter
  Atrial beating rates of approximately 300 bpm

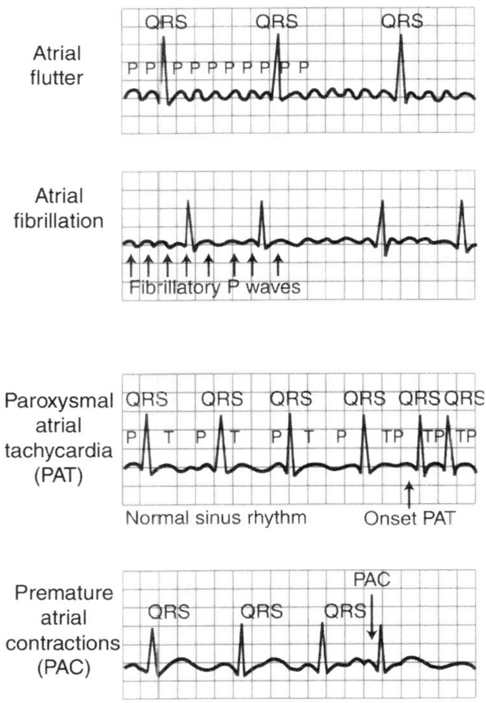

Figure 13.4 Atrial arrhythmias. (From Porth, C.M., *Pathophysiology: Concepts of Altered Health States*, 5th ed., Lippincott, Philadelphia, 1998. With permission.)

- Atrial fibrillation
  Uncoordinated contraction of atria

Filling of the ventricles occurs mainly as a passive process; contraction of the atria is necessary only to prime the ventricles or to "top them off" for contraction. As a result individuals may survive for months or even years with atrial fibrillation although with a somewhat reduced (approximately 25%) efficiency of heart pumping.

Since the maximum rate at which the AV node can conduct impulses is approximately 180 bpm, the ventricles are somewhat "protected" from the high beating rates of the atria during atrial flutter. However, the ventricles are not protected from very high beating rates if the arrhythmia arises in the ventricles.

Ventricular arrhythmia (Figure 13.5)

- *Ventricular premature beats*
  One of the most common types of arrhythmia
  Can progress into ventricular tachycardia or fibrillation
- *Ventricular tachycardia*
  Excessive ventricular contraction rates
  Can have marked effects on cardiac output
- *Ventricular fibrillation*
  The most serious cardiac arrhythmia
  Characterized by a complete loss of ventricular coordination
  Cardiac output falls to zero
  Rapid death will ensue if not treated (see Table 13.1)

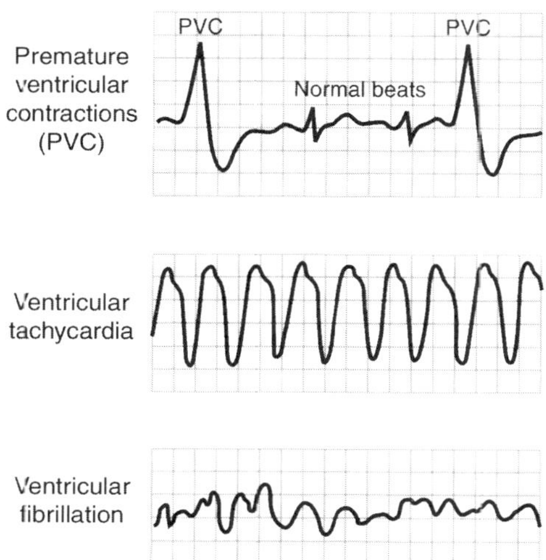

Figure 13.5 Ventricular arrhythmias. (From Porth, C.M., *Pathophysiology: Concepts of Altered Health States*, 5th ed., Lippincott, Philadelphia, 1998. With permission.)

Table 13.1 Treatment of Ventricular Fibrillation

Ventricular fibrillation is a life-threatening condition that must be treated immediately. The sequence for the treatment of acute ventricular fibrillation in order of preference is as follows:

DC-cardioversion — External electrical stimulation of heart puts the myocardium into a refractory state for a few seconds. When the heart begins to beat again normal pacing may resume.

Intravenous lidocaine or *procainamide* — Sodium channel blockers exert "local anesthetic-like" effects on the myocardium. They reduce automaticity and alter the threshold for excitability.

Arrhythmias that increase or decrease heart rate will directly affect cardiac output as cardiac output = heart rate × stroke volume. (Stroke Volume = the amount of blood pumped by one ventricle during one contraction) Up to a point, as heart rate increases, cardiac output will also increase. However, at very fast ventricular beating rates, the ventricles may be contracting so quickly that they do not have time to fill properly with blood. As a result cardiac output will now fall.

Heart block (Figure 13.6)

- Abnormal conduction of impulses by the bundle of His (AV bundle)
- Affects conduction of impulses between atria and ventricles
- May be a delay or complete block of impulse conduction

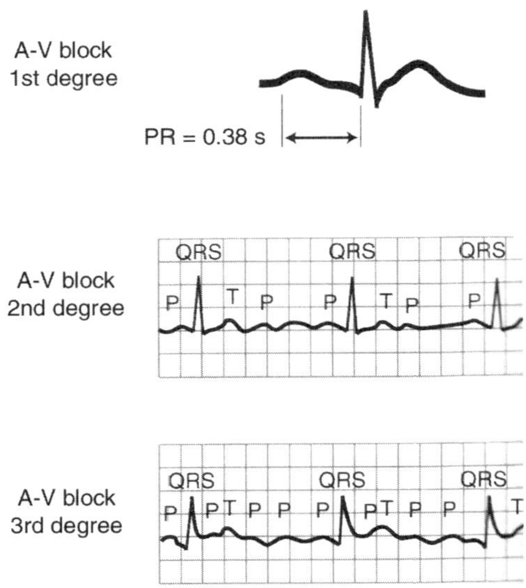

Figure 13.6 Degrees of heart block. (From Porth, C.M., *Pathophysiology: Concepts of Altered Health States*, 5th ed., Lippincott, Philadelphia, 1998. With permission.)

- May arise from ischemia, injury or inflammation of AV bundle
- Excessive stimulation or certain drugs might also block conduction through the AV bundle

Heart block may be classified as *first degree, second degree,* or *third degree* depending on the severity of the block.

1. First-degree heart block
   - All impulses are conducted between atria and ventricles but at a slowed rate.
   - Presents on the ECG as a prolonged P-Q interval.
2. Second-degree heart block
   - Some impulses are conducted to the ventricles, some are not.
   - Presents on the ECG as occasional missing QRS complexes.
   - Missing beats are called "dropped beats."
3. Third-degree heart block
   - No impulses are conducted from the atria to the ventricles.
   - Also called "complete heart block."
   - Heart will stop beating unless secondary pacemakers begin to function.

Stokes–Adams syndrome — Complete heart block that occurs suddenly and then subsides. Often associated with transient ischemia of the conduction pathways.

Bundle branch block — Defective conduction in left or right bundle branches that carry impulses through the ventricular septum. May significantly prolong ventricular depolarization.

Question

Which cardiac arrhythmias would have the greatest effect on cardiac output?

Diagnosis of arrhythmia

A number of techniques may be utilized to diagnose the presence of a cardiac arrhythmia (see Table 13.2). Since the occurrence of an arrhythmia may be episodic, long-term monitoring of cardiac electrophysiology may be necessary in certain patients.

Rationale for the treatment of cardiac arrhythmia

Cardiac arrhythmia may be treated by reducing abnormal automaticity of ectopic pacemakers or by reducing the occurrence of re-entry impulses by

Table 13.2 Diagnosis of Cardiac Arrhythmia

Resting ECG — Done only for a limited time and may miss episodes of arrhythmia
Exercise stress-testing with ECG — Exercise may induce changes in the ECG that are indicative of underlying conduction abnormalities or arrhythmia
Signal-averaged ECG — Special computerized ECG that averages QRS complexes to detect electrical changes in the heart that predispose a person to arrhythmia and fibrillation
Holter monitoring — Ambulatory, portable ECG monitor that can record the electrical activity of the heart for 1 to 2 days at a time to detect episodes of arrhythmia
Cardiac catheterization — Invasive techniques in which electrodes are inserted directly into the heart to measure electrical activity

increasing the duration of the refractory period of the myocardium. In effect, further reducing cardiac conduction may convert a one-way conduction block to a two-way conduction block and thus prevent re-entry impulses from initiating second depolarizations. Antiarrhythmic drugs are generally classified into four distinct classes based on their mechanism of action.

Treatment of cardiac arrhythmia

Pharmacologic treatment

Because of their marked effects on cardiac electrophysiology, *all* of the drugs used to treat cardiac arrhythmias can also cause cardiac arrhythmias (see Table 13.3).

Class I antiarrhythmic drugs
- Block voltage-gated sodium channels, local-anesthetic-like actions on cardiac cells
- Decrease "automaticity" and reduce conduction velocity
- Used for atrial and ventricular arrhythmias
- Examples: *quinidine, procainamide, lidocaine*

Class II antiarrhythmic drugs
- β-Adrenoreceptor antagonists that block β-adrenergic receptors in the heart
- Blunt the effects of the sympathetic nervous system on the heart
- Increase the refractory period of the AV node
- Example: *propranolol*

Class III antiarrhythmic drugs
- Increase the refractory period and extend overall duration of the cardiac action potential
- Examples: *amiodarone, sotalol*

Class IV antiarrhythmic drugs
- Block voltage-gated calcium channels
- Slow depolarization of pacemakers and conduction through AV node
- Examples: *verapamil, diltiazem*

Table 13.3 Adverse Effects of Drugs Used to Treat Arrhythmia

Class I Drugs — Quinidine, disopyramide
Urinary retention, constipation, blurred vision
Rare hypersensitivity reactions (may be severe)
Arrhythmia due to overly slow conduction
Lidocaine
Used intravenously only
Central nervous system effects, drowsiness, disorientation, convulsions
Class II Drugs — Propranolol
Bronchospasm, reduced cardiac output, worsened heart block
Class II Drugs — Amiodarone
Very long half-life (up to 100 days)
Numerous possible ill effects such as hypersensitivity, thyroid abnormalities, pulmonary fibrosis, corneal effects, gastrointestinal disturbances, potentially life-threatening arrhythmias
Class IV Drugs — Verapamil, diltiazem
Markedly decreased cardiac output and conduction that may precipitate heart failure
Hypotension, heart block

Nonpharmacologic treatment of arrhythmia

1. Surgical or electrical ablation of accessory conduction pathways that might be involved in conduction of abnormal impulses.
2. Implantable cardioverter-defibrillator (ICD) — A device that automatically detects the occurrence of potentially life-threatening arrhythmias and automatically treats them through electrical defibrillation.
3. Implantable pacemakers — May be used temporarily or permanently to pace the rate and rhythm of the heart in instances where the normal pacemaker system of the heart has failed.

chapter fourteen

Disorders of the respiratory system

Study objectives

- Describe the general symptoms of respiratory disease.
- List the major organisms responsible for the common cold.
- Discuss the key features of an influenza infection. How do endemics, epidemics and pandemics differ?
- Describe the drugs that are currently available for treating influenza. How are they similar? How do they differ?
- Compare and contrast typical and atypical pneumonia.
- List specific organisms that are associated with hospital-acquired and community-acquired pneumonia.
- List populations that are most at risk for pneumonia.
- Discuss the etiology and manifestations of tuberculosis. How can it be treated?
- Discuss the possible etiology of bronchial asthma. What are some potential asthma triggers?
- Compare and contrast the "early" and "late" phases of asthma in terms of their effects on the respiratory passages and clinical manifestations.
- Describe how asthma attacks are classified based on frequency and severity of attacks.
- Describe the various means by which asthma might be treated.
- Compare and contrast chronic bronchitis and emphysema in terms of etiology and clinical manifestations.
- Describe the different types of pneumothorax that might occur. What might cause each?
- Define atelectasis. What are the various types that might occur? What might cause each?
- Discuss the etiology of cystic fibrosis. What are the major clinical manifestations? Why does each occur?

- What is adult respiratory distress syndrome? How does it differ from respiratory distress syndrome in the newborn?
- List some possible causes of interstitial lung disease. How do interstitial lung diseases differ from diseases such as emphysema and chronic bronchitis?
- List some possible causes of respiratory failure. What are the major manifestations of respiratory failure?

Introduction

Respiratory illness is a major cause of mortality and morbidity in the United States. Respiratory structures such as the airways, alveoli and pleural membranes may all be affected by various disease processes. These respiratory diseases include infections such as pneumonia and tuberculosis, as well as *obstructive* disorders such as asthma, bronchitis and emphysema that obstruct airflow into and out of the lungs. Other conditions such as pneumothorax, atelectasis, respiratory distress syndrome and cystic fibrosis are classified as *restrictive* disorders, as they limit normal expansion of the lungs. Pulmonary function may also be affected by exposure to inhaled particles or by the growth of cancers. General symptoms of respiratory disease are listed in Table 14.1.

Table 14.1 General Symptoms of Respiratory Disease

Hypoxia — Decreased levels of oxygen in the tissues
Hypoxemia — Decreased levels of oxygen in arterial blood
Hypercapnia — Increased levels of CO_2 in the blood
Hypocapnia — Decreased levels of CO_2 in the blood
Dyspnea — Difficulty breathing
Tachypnea — Rapid rate of breathing
Cyanosis — Bluish discoloration of skin and mucous membranes due to poor oxygenation of the blood
Hemoptysis — Blood in the sputum

Respiratory infections

Infections of the respiratory tract can occur in the upper or lower respiratory tract, or both. Organisms capable of infecting respiratory structures include bacteria, viruses and fungi. Depending on the organism and extent of infection, the manifestations can range from mild to severe and even life-threatening.

Infections of the upper respiratory tract

The common cold

The majority of upper respiratory tract infections are caused by viruses. The most common viral pathogens for the "common cold" are *rhinovirus, parainfluenza virus, respiratory syncytial virus, adenovirus* and *coronavirus.* These viruses tend to have seasonal variations in their peak incidence and are readily spread from person to person via respiratory secretions. They gain entry to the body through the nasal mucosa and the surfaces of the eye.

Manifestations of the common cold include:

- *Rhinitis* — Inflammation of the nasal mucosa
- *Sinusitis* — Inflammation of the sinus mucosa

- *Pharyngitis* — Inflammation of the pharynx and throat
- Headache
- Nasal discharge and congestion

Influenza

Influenza is a viral infection that can affect the upper or lower respiratory tract. Three distinct forms of influenza virus have been identified: A, B and C. Of these three variants, type A is the most common and causes the most serious illness. The influenza virus is a highly transmissible respiratory pathogen. Because the organism has a high tendency for genetic mutation, new variants of the virus are constantly arising in different places around the world. Serious *pandemics* of influenza are seen every 8 to 10 years as a result of this genetic mutation (see Table 14.2).

Table 14.2 Epidemiology of Influenza Infection

Endemic — Outbreak of disease in a particular population that occurs in a regular, predictable manner
Epidemic — Outbreak of disease affecting a large number of individuals in a population
Pandemic — Outbreak of disease that is worldwide

Symptoms of influenza infection:

- Headache
- Fever, chills
- Muscle aches
- Nasal discharge
- Unproductive cough
- Sore throat

Influenza infection can cause marked inflammation of the respiratory epithelium leading to acute tissue damage and a loss of ciliated cells that protect the respiratory passages from other organisms. As a result, influenza infection may lead to co-infection of the respiratory passages with bacteria. It is also possible for the influenza virus to infect the tissues of the lung itself to cause a *viral pneumonia*.

Treatment of influenza:

- Bed rest, fluids, warmth
- Antiviral drugs (see Table 14.3)
- Influenza vaccine — Provides protection against certain A and B influenza strains that are expected to be prevalent in a certain year. The vaccine must be updated and administered yearly to be effective but will not be effective against influenza strains not included in the vaccine. The influenza vaccine is particularly indicated in elderly people, in individuals weakened by other disease and in health-care workers.

Table 14.3 Drugs for Treating Influenza

Amantidine
Used orally or by aerosol administration
Effective only against type A influenza
Inhibits viral fusion, assembly and release from the infected host cell
Neuraminidase inhibitors (Zanamavir, Oseltamivir)
New drugs that can be used by inhalation (Zanamavir) or orally (Oseltamivir)
Effective against both type A and B influenza
Inhibits the activity of viral neuraminidase enzyme that is necessary for spread of the influenza virus

Infections of the lower respiratory tract

The respiratory tract is protected by a number of very effective defense mechanisms designed to keep infectious organisms and particulates from reaching the lungs (see Table 14.4). For an organism to reach the lower respiratory tract, the organism must be particularly virulent and present in very large number or the host defense barriers must be weakened. One factor that might weaken the respiratory defense barriers is cigarette smoking, which can paralyze the cilia lining the cells of the respiratory passages and impair removal of secretions, particles and microorganisms. The presence of a respiratory pathogen such as the cold or influenza virus may also cause an inflammatory reaction that impairs the defense barriers of the respiratory passages and opens an individual to infection by other respiratory pathogens.

Table 14.4 Defenses of the Respiratory System

Moist, mucus-covered surfaces — Trap particles and organisms
Cell surface IgA, lysosomes
Ciliated epithelium — Clears trapped particles and organisms from airway passages
Cough reflex and epiglottis — Prevents aspiration of particles and irritants into lower airways
Pulmonary macrophages — Phagocytize foreign particles and organisms in the alveolar spaces

Pneumonia

Pneumonia is a condition that involves inflammation of lower lung structures such as the alveoli or interstitial spaces. It may be caused by bacteria, viruses or parasites such as *pneumocystis carinii*. Despite advances in drug therapy, pneumonia is still the sixth leading cause of death in the United States (see Table 14.5). The prevalence and severity of pneumonia have been heightened in recent years due to the emergence of HIV as well as antibiotic resistance.[16] Pneumonia may be classified according to the pathogen that is responsible for the infection. There tend to be distinct organisms that cause pneumonia in the hospital setting vs. the community setting.[17]

Table 14.5 Individuals Most at Risk for Pneumonia
Elderly
Those with viral infection
Chronically ill
AIDS or immunosuppressed patients
Smokers
Patients with chronic respiratory disease

Classification of pneumonia:

1. Hospital acquired
   - Enteric Gram-negative organisms (*Escherichia coli, Pseudomonas aeruginosa, Staphylococcus aureus)*
2. Community acquired
   - *Streptococcus pneumoniae, Haemophilus pneumoniae, Mycoplasma pneumoniae,* Influenza

A second classification scheme for pneumonia is based on the specific structures of the lung that the organisms infect and includes *typical* and *atypical* pneumonia.

Typical pneumonia

- Usually bacterial in origin.
- Organisms replicate in the spaces of the alveoli.

Manifestations:

- Inflammation and fluid accumulation are seen in the alveoli.
- White cell infiltration and exudation that can been seen on chest radiographs.
- High fever, chest pain, chills, and malaise are present.
- Purulent sputum is present.
- Some degree of hypoxemia is present.

Atypical pneumonia

- Usually viral in origin.
- Organisms replicate in the spaces around the alveoli.

Manifestations:

- Milder symptoms than typical pneumonia.
- Lack of white cell infiltration in alveoli.
- Lack of fluid accumulation in the alveoli.
- Not usually evident on radiographs.
- May make the patient susceptible to bacterial pneumonia.

Opportunistic organisms

A number of organisms not commonly associated with respiratory illness in otherwise healthy individuals can cause severe respiratory infections and pneumonia in patients with HIV or those who are immunocompromised as a result of immune suppressive therapy. These organisms include mycobacteria, fungus (*Histoplasma)* and protozoa (*Pneumocystis carinii*). Treatment of these organisms requires specific drug therapy, and, in the case of protozoa and fungi, the organisms are very difficult to kill.

Treatment of pneumonia:

- Antibiotics if bacterial in origin. The health-care provider should consider the possibility that antibiotic-resistant organisms are present.
- Oxygen therapy for hypoxemia.
- A vaccine for *pneumococcal* pneumonia is currently available and highly effective. This vaccine should be considered in high-risk individuals.

Tuberculosis

Tuberculosis is an infectious disease caused by the organism *Mycobacterium tuberculosis*. Unlike most other bacteria, *M. tuberculosis* is surrounded by an outer capsule that makes the organism very resistant to destruction. *Mycobacterium tuberculosis* is primarily transmitted via the airborne route. Once in the lung tissues, the organism causes an inflammatory reaction as it is attacked first by polymorphonuclear leukocytes and later by macrophages. The primary lesion that results in the lung during tuberculosis infection is called the *Ghon's focus*. If the lesion also involves regional lymph nodes, it is termed a *Ghon's complex*. Necrosis of infected lung tissues may result in a cheesy appearance to the tissue that is referred to as a *caseous necrosis*. *Liquefaction* of the necrotic lesions might also occur over time (see Chapter 1).

In an otherwise healthy individual, the immune system is usually able to contain the organism and over time will encapsulate it through *calcification* of the lesions. These calcified Ghon's complexes are readily visualized by chest radiograph for the remainder of the patient's life (see Table 14.6). Because live *M. tuberculosis* is often found within these encapsulations, impairment of immune function in the infected individual may lead to *reactivation* of the primary infection.

Table 14.6 Testing for Tuberculosis

Mantoux test — Intradermal test for reaction against the tuberculin purified protein derivative standard (PPDS)
Acid-fast staining of sputum cultures to visualize *M. tuberculosis*
Chest radiograph to identify Ghon's complex

Manifestations of primary tuberculosis:

- Productive, prolonged cough
- Chest pain, *hemoptysis*
- Chill, fever, night sweats
- Anorexia, weight loss

Treatment of tuberculosis: Despite a continuous decline in the incidence of tuberculosis in the decades preceding the 1980s, since 1985 there has been a steady increase in the worldwide incidence of tuberculosis. A major contributing factor to this resurgence of tuberculosis has been the spread of HIV. *Mycobacterium tuberculosis* can be a opportunistic organism that infects AIDS patients whose immune systems are weakened and inadequate to combat the organism. The rise of homelessness may also be a contributing factor to increased rates of tuberculosis in urban settings, as the organism thrives in the dark, dank environments in which homeless people sometimes dwell. Management of tuberculosis often requires prolonged treatment with powerful antimycobacterial drugs (see Table 14.7). Unfortunately, in recent years the treatment of tuberculosis has been complicated by the rise of organisms that are resistant to one or more of the commonly used antitubercular agents.[16] In cases of multidrug-resistant tuberculosis, mortality can be on then order of 70 to 90%. Factors that affect immune function such as proper nutrition and management of other diseases are also essential for successful treatment of tuberculosis.

Table 14.7 Drugs for the Treatment of Tuberculosis

Isoniazid
Active only against mycobacteria
Used orally, mechanism of action is uncertain
Resistance can result from reduced penetration of the drug into the organism
Rifampicin
Used orally, it is highly active at inhibiting the activity of RNA polymerase in mycobacteria
Inducer of liver enzymes and thus may affect metabolism of other liver-metabolized drugs
Resistance can emerge rapidly
Ethambutol
Used orally to inhibit the growth of mycobacteria
Mechanism of action is uncertain
Resistance can develop rapidly

Question

What are some factors that might contribute to tuberculosis drug resistance?

Obstructive respiratory disorders

Bronchial asthma

Asthma is a condition characterized by reversible bronchospasm and chronic inflammation of airway passages. The incidence of asthma has been steadily increasing in recent years. Although the exact etiology is still uncertain, there appears to be a definite genetic predisposition to the development of asthma. A key component of asthma appears to be airway "hyperreactivity" in affected individuals. Exposure to certain "triggers" can induce marked bronchospasm and airway inflammation in susceptible patients (see Tables 14.8 and 14.9). Individuals with asthma appear to produce large amounts of the antibody IgE that attach to the *mast cells* present in many tissues. Exposure to a trigger such as pollen will result in the allergen-binding mast cell-bound IgE, which in turn causes the release of inflammatory mediators such as *histamine, leukotrienes* and *eosinophilic chemotactic factor.* The response of a patient with asthma to these triggers can be divided into an "early phase" and a "late phase."

Table 14.8 Some Potential Asthma Triggers

Allergens — Pollen, pet dander, fungi, dust mites
Cold air
Pollutants
Cigarette smoke
Strong emotions
Exercise
Respiratory tract infections

Table 14.9 Clinical Classification of Asthma

Mild intermittent — Attacks occur 2 times per week or less
Mild persistent — Attacks occur more than 2 times per week
Moderate persistent — Attacks occur daily or almost daily and are severe enough to affect activity
Severe persistent — Attacks are very frequent and persist for a long period of time; attacks severely limit activity

Question

What are some of the factors that might be responsible for the increased occurrence of asthma in recent years?

Early phase of asthma: The early phase of asthma is characterized by marked constriction of bronchial airways and bronchospasm that is accompanied by edema of the airways and the production of excess mucus. The bronchospasm that occurs may be the result of the increased release of certain inflammatory mediators such as histamine, prostaglandins and bradykinin that, in the early stages of asthmatic response, promote bronchoconstriction rather than inflammation.

Late phase of asthma: The late phase of asthma can occur several hours after the initial onset of symptoms and manifests mainly as an inflammatory response. The primary mediators of inflammation during the asthmatic response are the white blood cells *eosinophils* that stimulate mast cell degranulation and release substances that attract other white cells to the area. Subsequent infiltration of the airway tissues with white blood cells such as neutrophils and lymphocytes also contributes to the overall inflammatory response of the late phase of asthma.

Manifestations of asthma (see Table 14.10):

- Coughing, wheezing
- Difficulty breathing
- Rapid, shallow breathing
- Increased respiratory rate
- Excess mucus production
- Barrel chest due to trapping of air in the lungs
- Significant anxiety

Complications of asthma: Possible complications of asthma can include the occurrence of *status asthmaticus,* which is a life-threatening condition of prolonged bronchospasm that is often not responsive to drug therapy. *Pneumothorax* is also a possible consequence as a result of lung pressure increases

Table 14.10 Staging of the Severity of an Acute Asthma Attack[18]

Stage I (mild)
Mild dyspnea
Diffuse wheezing
Adequate air exchange
Stage II (moderate)
Respiratory distress at rest
Marked wheezing
Stage III (severe)
Marked respiratory distress
Cyanosis
Marked wheezing or absence of breath sounds
Stage IV (respiratory failure)
Severe respiratory distress, lethargy, confusion, prominent pulsus paradoxus

Source: Berkow, R., Ed., *The Merck Manual*, 16th ed., Merck Research Laboratories, Rahway, NJ, 1992, 648. With permission.

that can result from the extreme difficulty involved in expiration during a prolonged asthma attack. Marked hypoxemia and acidosis might also occur and can result in overall respiratory failure.

Treatment of asthma: The appropriate drug treatment regimen for asthma is based on the frequency and severity of the asthma attacks and may include the following:

1. Avoidance of triggers, and allergens. Improved ventilation of the living spaces, use of air conditioning.
2. *Bronchodilators* (examples: albuterol, terbutaline) — Short acting β-*adrenergic* receptor activators. May be administered as needed in the form of a nebulizer solution using a metered dispenser or may be given subcutaneously. These drugs block bronchoconstriction but *do not* prevent the inflammatory response.
3. *Xanthine drugs* (example: theophylline) — Cause bronchodilation but may also inhibit the late phase of asthma. These drugs are often used orally as second-line agents in combination with other asthma therapies such as steroids. Drug like theophylline can have significant central nervous system, cardiovascular and gastrointestinal side effects that limit their overall usefulness.
4. *Anti-inflammatory drugs* (corticosteroids) — Used orally or by inhalation to blunt the inflammatory response of asthma. The most significant unwanted effects occur with long-term oral use of corticosteroids and may include immunosuppression, increased susceptibility to infection, osteoporosis and effects on other hormones such as the glucocorticoids.
5. *Cromolyn sodium* — Anti-inflammatory agent that blocks both the early and late phase of asthma. The mechanism of action is unclear but may involve mast cell function or responsiveness to allergens.
6. *Leukotriene modifiers* (example: Zafirlukast) — New class of agents that blocks the synthesis of the key inflammatory mediators, leukotrienes.

Bronchitis

Bronchitis is an obstructive respiratory disease that may occur in both acute and chronic forms.

Acute bronchitis: Inflammation of the bronchial passages most commonly caused by infection with bacteria or viruses. Acute bronchitis is generally a self-limiting condition in healthy individuals but can have much more severe consequences in individuals who are weakened with other illness or who are immunocompromised. Symptoms of acute bronchitis often include productive cough, dyspnea and possible fever.

Chronic bronchitis: Chronic bronchitis is a chronic obstructive pulmonary disease that is most frequently associated with cigarette smoking (approximately 90% of cases). Chronic bronchitis may also be caused by prolonged exposure to inhaled particulates such as coal dust or other pollutants. The disease is characterized by excess mucus production in the lower respiratory tract. This mucus accumulation can impair function of the ciliated epithelium and lining of the respiratory tract and prevent the clearing of debris and organisms. As a result, patients with chronic bronchitis often suffer repeated bouts of respiratory infection. Chronic bronchitis sufferers are often referred to as "blue bloaters" as a result of the cyanosis and peripheral edema that is often present.

Manifestations of chronic bronchitis:

- Productive, chronic cough
- Production of purulent sputum
- Frequent respiratory infections
- Dyspnea
- Hypoxia, cyanosis
- Symptoms of *cor pulmonale* (see Chapter 12)
- Fluid accumulation in later stages

Treatment of chronic bronchitis:

1. Cessation of smoking or exposure to irritants
2. Bronchodilators to open airway passages
3. Expectorants to loosen mucus
4. Anti-inflammatories to relieve airway inflammation and reduce mucus secretion
5. Prophylactic antibiotics for respiratory infections
6. Oxygen therapy

Emphysema

Emphysema is a respiratory disease that is characterized by destruction and permanent enlargement of terminal bronchioles and alveolar air sacs (see Figure 14.1). Well over 95% of all patients with emphysema were chronic cigarette smokers. Although the exact etiology of emphysema is still uncertain, it appears that chronic exposure to cigarette smoke causes chronic inflammation of the alveolar airways, which results in infiltration by lymphocytes and macrophages. Excess release of protease enzymes such as trypsin from lung tissues and leukocytes can digest and destroy the elastic walls of the alveoli. Alveolar air sacs become enlarged and distended as their structure is affected and their elasticity lost. Levels of a protective enzyme *α-1-antitrypsin* have been shown to be lacking in certain individuals who are chronic cigarette smokers. This enzyme inactivates destructive protease enzymes in lung tissue. In fact, a rare form of emphysema occurs in individuals who are not cigarette smokers but who have a genetic lack of α-1-antitrypsin.

Manifestations of emphysema: The major physiologic changes seen in emphysema are a loss of alveolar (lung) elasticity and a decrease in the overall surface area for gas exchange within the lungs. Manifestations include the following (see Table 14.11):

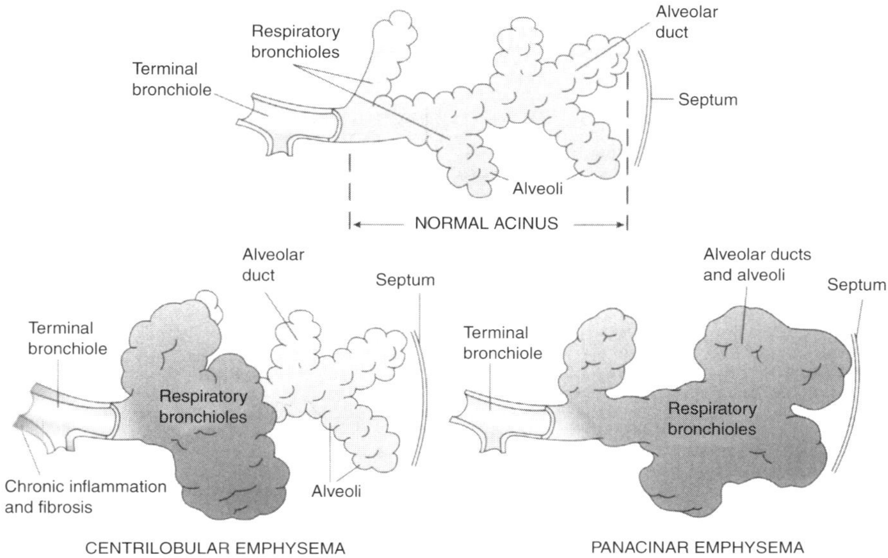

Figure 14.1 Types of emphysema. (From Porth, C.M., *Pathophysiology: Concepts of Altered Health States*, 5th ed., Lippincott, Philadelphia, 1998. With permission.)

Table 14.11 Comparison of Symptoms for Chronic Bronchitis and Emphysema

Chronic bronchitis	Emphysema
Mild dyspnea	Dyspnea that may be severe
Productive cough	Dry or no cough
Cyanosis common	Cyanosis rare
Respiratory infection common	Infrequent infections
Onset usually after 40 years of age	Onset usually after 50 years of age
History of cigarette smoking	History of cigarette smoking
Cor pulmonale common	Cor pulmonale in terminal stages

- Tachypnea (increased respiratory rate): Because the increased respiratory rate in these individuals is effective in maintaining arterial blood gases, one does not usually see hypoxia or cyanosis until the end stages of the disease. Patients with emphysema are often referred to as "pink puffers" because of their high respiratory rates and lack of obvious cyanosis.
- Dyspnea
- Barrel chest from prolonged expiration
- Lack of purulent sputum
- Possible long-term consequences, including *cor pulmonale*, respiratory failure

Restrictive pulmonary disorders

Pneumothorax (see Figure 14.2)

Pneumothorax is the entry of air into the pleural cavity in which the lungs reside. In order for normal lung expansion to occur, there must be a negative pressure within the pleural cavity with respect to atmospheric pressure outside the pleural cavity. The inside of the pleural cavity is essentially a vacuum and when air enters the pleural cavity the negative pressure is lost and the lungs collapse. Because each lung sits in a separate pleural cavity, pneumothorax of one plural cavity will not cause collapse of the other lung.

Types of pneumothorax:

1. Open or communicating pneumothorax
   - Usually involves a traumatic chest wound.
   - Air enters the pleural cavity from the atmosphere.
   - The lung collapses due to equilibration of pressure within the pleural cavity with atmospheric pressure.
2. Closed or spontaneous pneumothorax
   - Occurs when air "leaks" from the lungs into the pleural cavity.
   - May be caused by lung cancer, rupture, pulmonary disease.
   - The increased plural pressure prevents lung expansion during inspiration and the lung remains collapsed.

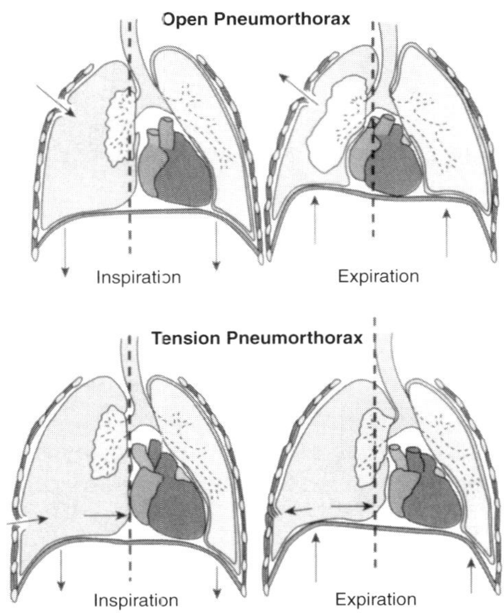

Figure 14.2 Pneumothorax. (From Porth, C.M., *Pathophysiology: Concepts of Altered Health States*, 5th ed., Lippincott, Philadelphia, 1998. With permission.)

3. Tension pneumothorax
   - A condition in which there is a one-way movement of air into but not out of the pleural cavity.
   - May involve a hole or wound to the pleural cavity that allows air to enter and the lung to collapse. Upon expiration, the hole or opening closes, which prevents the movement of air back out of the pleural cavity.
   - A life-threatening condition because pressure in the pleural cavity continues to increase and may result in further lung compression or compression of large blood vessels in the thorax or the heart.

Manifestations of pneumothorax:

- Tachypnea, dyspnea
- Chest pain
- Possible compression of thoracic blood vessels and heart, especially with tension pneumothorax

Treatment of pneumothorax:

- Removal of air from the pleural cavity with a needle or chest tube
- Repair of trauma and closure of opening into pleural cavity

Atelectasis

Atelectasis is a condition in which there is incomplete expansion of lung tissues due to blockage of the airways or compression of the alveolar sacs.

Types of atelectasis:

1. Absorption atelectasis
   - Results when the bronchial passages are blocked with mucus, tumors or edema
   - May occur with conditions such as chronic bronchitis or *cystic fibrosis* (see below) in which there is the accumulation of excess mucus in the respiratory passages
2. Compression atelectasis
   - Occurs when lung tissue is compressed externally by air, blood, fluids or a tumor

Manifestations of atelectasis:

- Dyspnea, cough.
- Reduced gas exchange. The effects of atelectasis on gas exchange will depend on the amount of lung tissue that is prevented from expanding.
- Shunting of blood to areas of the lungs that are inflated. The *ventilation–perfusion coupling* ability of the lungs will help ensure that blood is directed to areas of the lungs where gas exchange can still occur.

Treatment of atelectasis:

- Removal of airway blockage
- Removal of air, blood, fluids, tumors, etc. that are compressing lung tissues

Bronchiectasis

Bronchiectasis is a condition that results from prolonged injury or inflammation of respiratory airways and bronchioles. It is characterized by abnormal dilation of the bronchus or bronchi. It is most frequently associated with chronic respiratory disease, infections, cystic fibrosis, tumor growth or exposure to respiratory toxins. The major manifestations of bronchiectasis are impaired ventilation of the alveoli, chronic inflammation and possible fibrosis of the areas.

Cystic fibrosis

Cystic fibrosis is a genetic disorder that affects function of exocrine glands throughout the body. The disorder is an autosomal recessive condition caused by a defect in the gene that codes for a cell membrane–associated protein called the *transmembrane conductance protein*. This protein is involved in regulation of chloride transport across the cell membrane. Lack of this protein results in production of overly thick mucus that cannot be cleared from the respiratory passages and accumulates to form *mucous plugs*. The accumulated mucus also becomes a breeding ground for numerous respiratory pathogens. Over time, chronic infection and inflammation of respiratory tissues will lead to deterioration of lung function and eventual respiratory failure, which is the leading cause of death in these patients. Excess mucus may also be produced by cells of the gastrointestinal tract, leading to possible gastrointestinal blockage and impairment of digestion. Exocrine function of the pancreas is also affected by this disorder and can result in impaired digestion of nutrients as well as possible destruction of the pancreas.

Manifestations of cystic fibrosis:

- Thick, viscous mucus in the respiratory and gastrointestinal tract
- Frequent, serious respiratory infections
- Obstruction of respiratory passages
- Progressive deterioration of respiratory function
- Dyspnea, hypoxemia
- Respiratory failure
- Pancreatic destruction, diabetes
- Gastrointestinal blockage
- Poor nutrient digestion

Treatment of cystic fibrosis:

- Use of prophylactic antibiotics to prevent respiratory infections
- Frequent manual drainage of respiratory secretions

- *K^+-sparing diuretic (amiloride)*, which used in aerosolized form has been shown to improve mucociliary clearance in patients with cystic fibrosis
- Bronchodilators
- Inhaled corticosteroids for chronic inflammation
- Gene therapy — Possible that in the future the missing gene in cystic fibrosis may be introduced into affected cells using a viral vector
- Lung transplantation

Adult respiratory distress syndrome (ARDS)

ARDS is a syndrome associated with destruction of alveolar membranes and their related capillaries. It may occur as a result of direct injury to the lungs or as a result of dramatic decreases in blood flow to the lung ("shock lung," see Chapter 12). Some possible causes of ARDS are listed in Table 14.12.

Manifestations of ARDS:

- Dyspnea, tachypnea.
- Hypoxemia — CO_2 is significantly more water soluble than O_2 and can still be eliminated from the lungs via diffusion; as a result blood levels of oxygen are more affected by ARDS than CO_2. Hypocapnia may result.
- Infiltration of lung tissues with immune cells that release inflammatory mediators.
- Accumulation of fluids in alveoli and around alveolar spaces.
- Changes in blood pH due to altered blood levels of CO_2.
- Pulmonary fibrosis.
- Respiratory failure.

Treatment of ARDS:

- Oxygen therapy
- Anti-inflammatory drugs
- Diuretics to reduce edema
- Correction of acid–base balance

Table 14.12 Possible Causes of ARDS

Septicemia, uremia
Trauma
Near drowning
Inhalation of toxic gases or agents
Aspiration of gastric contents
Widespread pneumonia
Drug overdose
Systemic shock

Respiratory distress syndrome of the newborn

The etiology of newborn respiratory distress syndrome differs considerably from that of the adult disorder. Respiratory distress in the newborn is most commonly caused by a lack of surfactant in the lungs. Pulmonary surfactant is a mixture of lipids and proteins produced by Type II cells of the alveoli. A thin layer of surfactant covers the surfaces of the alveoli and provides surface tension that prevents the thin-walled alveoli from collapsing. Surfactant also moistens the alveolar surfaces to facilitate gas exchange. Respiratory distress syndrome of the newborn occurs most commonly in infants who are born prematurely and whose lungs have not developed to the point where they are producing adequate surfactant. Clinical manifestations become evident immediately at birth and can be rapidly fatal if not treated.

Manifestations of respiratory distress syndrome in the newborn:

- Rapid, shallow breathing
- Lung collapse
- Lung inflammation and damage
- Hypoxemia
- Nasal flaring, grunting upon inspiration

Treatment of respiratory distress syndrome in the newborn:

- Delay or prevention of premature delivery of infant if possible.
- Treatment of premature newborn with synthetic surfactant delivered directly into the lower respiratory tract. Exogenous surfactant will need to be supplied until the infant's lungs have matured to the point where they are producing their own surfactant.
- Mechanical ventilation.
- Injection of cortisol in the mother prior to delivery may significantly reduce the incidence of respiratory distress syndrome in premature infants. Cortisol has also been shown to stimulate activity of Type II cells.

Interstitial lung diseases

Interstitial lung diseases represent a number of restrictive disorders whose main characteristic is scarring and fibrosis of lung tissue. The result of extensive lung scarring is reduced lung compliance and overall decreased lung volumes. Many causes of interstitial lung disease involve occupational exposure to injurious substances such as coal dust ("black lung"), asbestos (asbestosis), silicone dust (silicosis), radiation, drugs or toxins (see Table 14.13). Chronic lung infections, pulmonary edema or tumors might also lead to scarring and fibrosis of lung tissue. However, the etiology of a significant percentage of interstitial lung disease remains unknown.

Manifestations of interstitial lung disease:

- Dyspnea, tachypnea
- Cough

Table 14.13 Possible Causes of Interstitial Lung Diseases

Exposure to injurious substances
Coal dust
Asbestos
Silicone dust
Talc
Organic dusts (hay, cotton, etc.)
Noxious gases
Radiation
Anticancer drugs
Infectious agents
Unknown causes
Sarcoidosis — An immune disorder that affects the lungs, skin and eyes
Connective tissue diseases

- Hypoxemia
- Clubbing of fingers due to chronic hypoxia
- Progressive deterioration of pulmonary function and possible respiratory failure

Treatment of interstitial lung diseases: Treatment options for these disorders are limited and mainly focus on removal of the injurious substances. Anti-inflammatory drugs may be of use in limiting damage from chronic inflammation. Oxygen therapy may be instituted in severe cases.

Respiratory failure

Respiratory failure is a condition that results when the lungs are no longer able to oxygenate the blood sufficiently or remove CO_2 from it. It may occur as the end result of chronic respiratory diseases or it may be an acute event caused by factors such as pneumothorax or opioid drug overdose (see Table 14.14).

Manifestations of respiratory failure:

- Hypoxemia
- Hypercapnia
- Ventilation–perfusion mismatch
- Cyanosis, possible but not always present
- Central nervous system symptoms — Slurred speech, confusion, impaired motor function
- Altered blood pH
- Initial tachycardia and increased cardiac output followed by bradycardia and decreased cardiac output

Table 14.14 Causes of Respiratory Failure

Acute
Pneumothorax
Drug overdose (opioids, sedatives)
Pleural effusion — Accumulation of fluids in the pleural cavity
Airway obstruction
Status asthmaticus
Inhalation of toxins or noxious gases
Chronic
Emphysema
Interstitial lung diseases
Cystic fibrosis
Spinal cord or brain injury
Congestive heart failure
Neuromuscular disorders — Muscular dystrophy, myasthenia gravis, amyotrophic lateral sclerosis
Pulmonary emboli
Diffuse pneumonia
Pulmonary edema

Treatment of respiratory failure:

- Bronchodilators
- Correction of blood pH
- Oxygen therapy
- Mechanical ventilation

chapter fifteen

Abnormalities of the kidney and urinary tract

Study objectives

- List the various functions performed by the kidneys.
- Describe the different methods one can use to assess renal function. What are the pros and cons of each of these?
- Discuss the various mechanisms the kidney uses to help regulate renal blood flow. How can these factors worsen the physiologic changes that accompany renal disease?
- List some possible causes of acute and chronic glomerulonephritis. How does glomerulonephritis differ from pyelonephritis?
- What are renal calculi? What are some factors that can contribute to their formation? What effects might they have on the kidney?
- List prerenal, intrarenal and postrenal causes of renal failure. List the major physiologic effects of renal failure on the various systems of the body. Why does each occur?
- Describe the principle of hemodialysis. What is the role of hemodialysis in renal failure? How does peritoneal dialysis differ from classic hemodialysis? What are the advantages and disadvantages of each type of dialysis?
- List possible causes of urine reflux and neurogenic bladder. What are the possible consequences of each on the kidney?

Introduction

The urinary system comprises the kidneys, excretory ducts (ureters, renal calyces and pelves), bladder and urethra. The kidneys are responsible for the production of urine. Urine produced by the kidneys is carried by the ureters to the bladder where it is stored. The urethra conveys urine from the bladder to the exterior for excretion.

Disorders of the kidney

The kidneys are essential excretory organs that remove the waste products of metabolism from the body. In addition to their role in excretion, the kidneys also function in regulation of blood pressure, blood volume and erythropoiesis (see Table 15.1). In order for the kidneys to function normally three things must occur. First, there must be adequate blood flow through the glomerular capillaries. Second, the glomerular capillaries, which selectively filter blood, must be intact. Normal glomeruli allow fluids and small solutes to be filtered into the renal tubules but not proteins or blood cells. Third, the tubules of the kidney must be able to reabsorb essential substances selectively from the filtrate while excreting other substances into the filtrate to be eliminated in the final urine.

Table 15.1 Functions of the Kidney

Excretion of metabolic wastes
Regulation of mineral and water balance
Release of renin that is important in regulation of blood pressure and blood volume
Release of *erythropoietin* in response to hypoxia; erythropoietin stimulates the production of red blood cells in the bone marrow

Renal regulation of blood flow

Specialized cells located in the walls of the afferent glomerular arterioles called *juxtaglomerular* cells are capable of monitoring blood flow through the renal arterioles. In response to a decrease in renal blood flow, these cells release the enzyme *renin* into the bloodstream. In the circulation, renin interacts with a circulating protein called *angiotensinogen* and enzymatically cleaves it to a new peptide called angiotensin I, which in turn is rapidly converted to angiotensin II by angiotensin-converting enzyme (ACE). ACE is found in the endothelial cells that line small blood vessels of the lungs.

Effects of angiotensin II:

- Powerful and rapid vasoconstriction of blood vessels
- Direct action on the kidney to enhance salt and water retention
- Causes the adrenal glands to release *aldosterone*, which in turn increases salt and water reabsorption by the kidney tubules

Evaluation of renal function

Measurement of the rate at which substances are "cleared" from the plasma can be a means of evaluating how effectively the kidneys are functioning. To be useful as a measure of renal clearance, the substance measured can only be filtered by the kidneys and not reabsorbed or secreted by the kidney tubules. The most widely used method of estimating renal clearance involves measuring the rate at which *creatinine* is eliminated into the urine over a set period of time. Creatinine is a by-product of skeletal muscle metabolism and is present in the plasma at relatively constant levels. The main drawback to the use of "creatinine clearance" to measure renal function is that any condition that increases skeletal muscle breakdown (sepsis, muscle injury or muscle disease, for example) will elevate levels of serum creatinine and invalidate the measure. A second substance that can be used to estimate renal clearance is *inulin*. Inulin is a polysaccharide that is administered intravenously to the patient and its elimination in the urine is measured over time. Inulin offers the advantage that it is not metabolized or formed anywhere in the body and is eliminated only through renal filtration. The disadvantage to inulin is that it is not an endogenous substance and must be administered intravenously.

Acute glomerulonephritis

- Inflammation of the glomerulus.
- Occurs most commonly 7 to 10 days following an infection with group A streptococcus. Trapping of antibody–antigen complexes in glomerular capillaries causes inflammation of the glomerulus and alters its selective permeability, allowing plasma proteins and blood cells to enter the kidney filtrate.
- The active inflammatory process draws white blood cells that may enhance the inflammatory process.
- May also be related to systemic conditions such as *lupus erythematosus* and *Berger's disease* where there are excess levels of circulating antibodies or antigen–antibody complexes.
- Glomerular damage may result and certain patients may develop rapidly progressing glomerulonephritis or chronic glomerulonephritis.

Rapidly progressing glomerulonephritis

- Occurs most commonly in individuals in their 50s and 60s.

- May be idiopathic in origin or the result of acute glomerulonephritis or *Goodpasture syndrome* (see box).
- Presents with rapidly developing inflammation of the glomeruli and dramatic decreases in *glomerular filtration rate* (see definition box).
- May lead to renal failure.

Goodpasture syndrome

A rare form of rapidly progressing glomerulonephritis caused by antibodies that are produced against cells of the glomerulus. Leads to extensive inflammation and damage of the glomeruli to the point where renal failure may occur.

Definition

Glomerular filtration rate = amount of fluid that filters into Bowman's capsule per unit time

---

Chronic glomerulonephritis

- Chronic inflammation of the glomeruli.
- Etiology may be diverse; many patients with chronic glomerulonephritis may have no history of acute renal disease.
- May be associated with chronic hypertension, diabetes mellitus.
- May remain asymptomatic for a number of years before symptoms of proteinuria, hematuria occur.
- Progressive loss of renal function occurs over a number of years leading to renal insufficiency and renal failure.

Manifestations of glomerulonephritis

- Proteinuria (appearance of protein in the urine, primarily albumin)
- Hematuria (appearance of blood in the urine)
- With chronic forms of glomerulonephritis, decreased urine volume and fluid retention may occur as renal insufficiency and renal failure develops.
- Hypertension is a possible consequence of reduced renal blood flow and activation of renin–angiotensin system.

Treatment of glomerulonephritis

- Antibiotic therapy if caused by bacterial infection
- Immunosuppressive drugs if autoimmune destruction of glomeruli is occurring
- Management of resulting edema, mineral imbalance and possible hypertension

Urinary tract infections

- Generally caused by bacteria
- May occur in any of the urinary tract structures
- Occurs most frequently in females as well as senior citizens of both sexes

Manifestations

- Painful urination
- Increased urgency and frequency of urination
- *Cystitis* — Inflammation of the bladder
- *Pyelonephritis* — Inflammation of the kidneys that may be acute or chronic; possible that *chronic pyelonephritis* may lead to scarring of kidney structures and possible loss of kidney function
- Fever that may also occur along with the presence of white blood cells in the urine
- Frequent urinary tract infections in a patient might indicate the presence of a urinary tract obstruction or urine reflux.

Treatment

- Appropriate antibiotics
- Surgical correction of obstruction or structural abnormality that might be causing urine retention

Renal calculi (kidney stones)

- Form mainly in the renal pelves or calyces, but can form anywhere in the kidneys
- Composed mainly of calcium salts, uric acid and cystine
- Although the exact etiology is unclear, predisposing factors include the following:
  - Dehydration
  - Changes in urine pH
  - Decreased urine production
  - Excess salt secretion

- Gout
- Obstruction of urine flow

Manifestations

- Many renal calculi are asymptomatic until they obstruct kidney structures such as the calyces or pelves (see Table 15.2).
- Severe pain that can result from obstruction
- Fever, chills
- Hematuria
- Gastrointestinal symptoms (nausea, vomiting)
- Urine obstruction
- Complications that may include damage to renal structures and acute renal failure

Treatment

- Preventative measures include increased fluid intake, acidification of the urine and reduction of serum uric acid levels.
- Surgical removal of stones.
- *Lithotripsy* — Ultrasonic destruction of stones. Fragmented stones may then pass naturally with the urine.

Table 15.2 Diagnosis of Renal Calculi

Measurement of stone-forming substances in blood and urine
Radiography
Ultrasound

Renal tumors

Tumors of the kidney may be either rare benign *adenomas* or, more commonly, malignant *renal cell carcinomas*. If benign adenomas arise, they tend to be small and usually not clinically significant. The prognosis for renal cell carcinomas depends upon the morphology of the cells involved and the extent of spread outside the kidney. Renal carcinomas may metastasize to the lymphatics, liver, lungs and bone marrow.

Manifestations

- Hematuria
- Flank pain
- Weight loss
- Many renal tumors asymptomatic until the tumor is of advanced size and begins to disrupt renal structures
- Metastatic tumors that can occur with advanced disease

Treatment

- Chemotherapy, radiation therapy
- Surgical removal of tumors

Wilm's tumor (nephroblastoma)

Rare malignant tumor that arises in infants and children. The tumor presents with unique histology that may resemble embryonic kidney. Tumor can metastasize rapidly.

Polycystic kidney disease

Polycystic kidney disease is a hereditary disorder that can have an *autosomal dominant* (adult form) or *autosomal recessive* (childhood form) pattern of inheritance. Cysts develop in both kidneys and gradually increase in size. As normal kidney tissue is destroyed by the enlarging cysts, there is a progressive loss of renal function that may culminate in renal failure. The recessive form of the disease may cause renal failure in childhood while the dominant form progresses more slowly and generally does not lead to renal failure until patients enter their 60s or 70s.

Manifestations

- Grossly enlarged kidneys
- Hypertension from activation of the renin–angiotensin system
- Renal insufficiency leading to renal failure
- Pain in the flanks
- Frequent infections

Treatment

- Management of renal insufficiency and renal failure with dialysis
- Management of hypertension; patients may be at particular risk for aneurysms and cerebral hemorrhage
- Renal transplantation
- Antibiotics for frequent infections

Renal failure

Renal failure refers to a significant loss of renal function in both kidneys to the point where less than 10 to 20% of normal GFR remains. Renal failure may occur as an acute and rapidly progressing process or may

Table 15.3 Causes of Acute Renal Failure

Prerenal failure
Caused by impaired or reduced blood flow to the kidney
Possible causes: shock, hypotension, anaphylaxis, sepsis
Unless blood flow and oxygen delivery are restored permanent damage to the kidney will result
Intrarenal failure
Results from acute damage to renal structures
Possible causes: acute glomerulonephritis, pyelonephritis
May also result from *acute tubular necrosis* (ATN), which is damage of kidney structure from exposure to toxins, solvents, drugs and heavy metals; ATN is the most common cause of acute renal failure
Postrenal failure
Results from conditions that block urine outflow
Possible causes: obstruction of urine outflow by calculi, tumors, prostatic hypertrophy

present as a chronic form in which there is a progressive loss of renal function over a number of years. Possible causes of renal failure are listed in Table 15.3.

Acute renal failure

- Abrupt decrease in renal function.
- The possible causes of acute renal failure are shown in Table 15.3. These causes of acute renal failure may be *prerenal, intrarenal* or *postrenal* in nature. Acute renal failure is often reversible so long as permanent injury to the kidney has not occurred.

Manifestations

- *Oliguria* (reduced urine output)
- Possible edema and fluid retention
- Elevated blood urea nitrogen levels (BUN) and serum creatinine
- Alterations in serum electrolytes

Treatment

- Prevention of acute renal failure through support of blood pressure and blood volume
- Correction of fluid and electrolyte imbalances
- *Dialysis*, which may be employed while the kidneys are in the recovery phase
- Low protein, high carbohydrate diet to minimize the formation of nitrogenous wastes

Table 15.4 Stages of Chronic Renal Failure

Diminished renal reserve — GFR decreased to 35 to 50% of normal
Renal insufficiency — GFR decreased to 20 to 35% of normal
Renal failure — GFR reduced to less than 20% of normal
End-Stage Renal Disease — GFR is less than 5% of normal

Chronic renal failure

Chronic renal failure is the end result of progressive kidney damage and loss of function. Chronic renal failure is often classified into four progressive stages based on the loss of GFR (see Table 15.4). Some of the possible causes of chronic renal failure include the following:

- Chronic glomerulonephritis
- Chronic infections
- Renal obstruction
- Exposure to toxic chemicals, toxins or drugs (see aminoglycoside antibiotics and nephrotoxicity box)
- Diabetes
- Hypertension
- *Nephrosclerosis* (atherosclerosis of the renal artery)

Aminoglycoside antibiotics and nephrotoxicity

The aminoglycoside antibiotics are a widely used group of drugs that include agents such as streptomycin, gentamicin and kanamycin. The aminoglycosides can be nephrotoxic under certain conditions. Aminoglycoside toxicity is most likely to occur in elderly people, those with renal insufficiency or with chronic use. Concurrent use of loop diuretics may also compound the adverse renal effects of the aminoglycosides.

Manifestations

Because the kidneys play such an essential role in a number of physiologic processes, renal failure is a multisystem disease. The kidneys have a tremendous reserve capacity for function and as a result overt symptoms generally do occur until renal insufficiency is present. The effects of chronic renal failure on the various systems of the body are detailed in Table 15.5.

Vicious cycle of chronic renal failure

There are several physiologic adaptations that occur in the kidneys in response to chronic renal failure:

- Increased renal blood flow and GFR in functional nephrons
- Hypertrophy of functional nephrons

In the short term these adaptations may be beneficial, but in the long term the increased pressure in the kidneys and increased oxygen demand can further damage the nephrons and worsen renal failure.

Table 15.5 Effects of Chronic Renal Failure on Various Systems of the Body

System	Effect	Cause
Body fluids	Polyuria	Inability to concentrate urine
	Metabolic acidosis	Reduced H^+ excretion
	Abnormal levels of Na^+, K^+, Ca^{2+}, PO_4^-	Loss of tubular function
Hematologic	Anemia, excess bleeding	Impaired erythropoietin
Cardiovascular	Hypertension, edema	Activation of renin–angiotensin system
Gastrointestinal tract	Anorexia, nausea	Accumulation of metabolic wastes
Neurologic	Uremic encephalopathy	Accumulation of ammonia and nitrogenous waste
Musculoskeletal	Muscle and bone weakness ("Renal Osteodystrophy")	Loss of calcium and minerals

Treatment

- Careful management of fluids and electrolytes
- Prudent use of diuretics
- Careful dietary management; restriction of dietary protein intake
- Recombinant erythropoietin to treat anemia
- Renal dialysis (see Figure 15.1, and hemodialysis box)
- Renal transplantation

Hemodialysis

Hemodialysis is a procedure in which an "artificial kidney" machine takes the place of the patient's own failing kidneys. Using an indwelling catheter, blood is withdrawn from the patient and passed though a chamber containing a dialysis membrane and clean dialysate solution. Waste products that are in high concentration in the patient's blood diffuse across the dialysate membrane and into the dialysate solution. The cleaned blood is then returned to the patient via a second catheter. Complications to hemodialysis can include risk of infection, hypotension and electrolyte imbalance. Patients receiving hemodialysis must undergo the procedure several times per week for 3 to 6 hours per treatment. Newer high flux dialysate membranes and improved dialysate solutions have reduced the time of each dialysis session by 1 to 2 hours.

An alternative to classic hemodialysis is a technique called peritoneal dialysis. With this technique a "permanent" catheter is implanted into the peritoneal cavity. A clean dialysate solution is introduced through this catheter into the peritoneal cavity and the patient's own peritoneum (the membrane lining the abdominal cavity) is used as the dialyzing membrane. After a fixed period of time, usually 8 to 48 hours depending on the system and the frequency of dialysis, the used fluid is withdrawn. Complications of this technique may include infections from the catheter, hypotension, edema and metabolic abnormalities. Peritoneal dialysis does, however, offer the advantage that it may be performed in a patient's own home and overnight when the patient sleeps.

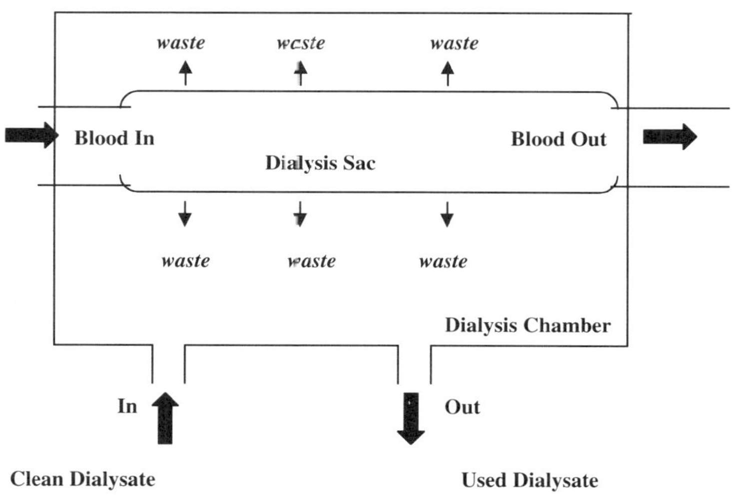

Figure 15.1 Principle of hemodialysis.

Disorders of the bladder and urethera

Urine reflux

Urine reflux is the backward flow of urine from the bladder into the ureters and kidneys (*vesicoureteral reflux*) or from the urethra into the bladder (*urethrovesical reflux*)

- Generally results from congenital abnormalities in the structure or location of the ureters or urethra.
- Patients often present with urine retention and recurrent urinary tract infections.
- Treatment may include antibiotic therapy and possible surgical correction of the structural abnormality.

Neurogenic bladder

- Bladder paralysis that occurs from interruption of nervous input to the muscles of the bladder wall.
- Patients are unable to voluntarily or involuntarily empty their bladder.
- Causes may include spinal cord trauma, polio, multiple sclerosis and tumors affecting spinal nerves.
- Manifestations include marked urine retention, frequent urinary tract infections and possible deterioration of renal function (post-renal failure).

chapter sixteen

Gastrointestinal disorders

Study objectives

- List general symptoms of gastrointestinal disease.
- Describe the various disorders that can affect the esophagus.
- Discuss peptic ulcer disease in terms of its cause(s), effects and treatment.
- Discuss the condition of irritable bowel syndrome. What may cause it?
- Compare and contrast Crohn's disease and ulcerative colitis in terms of their clinical similarities and differences. How might each be treated?
- How are cholelithiasis and cholecystitis related? What factors may contribute to cholelithiasis?
- How might one detect colorectal cancer? What are some factors that might predispose an individual to it? What are some of the possible pathophysiologic effects of colorectal cancer?
- What is diverticular disease? Why might it occur? Define diverticulitis.

Introduction

The gastrointestinal (G.I.) tract comprises the oral cavity, esophagus, stomach, small intestine (duodenum, jejunum, ileum) and large intestine (colon and rectum). Accessory organs such as the pancreas, liver and gallbladder play an important role in the digestive process. The process of digestion begins in the mouth with the mechanical grinding of food by the teeth. Saliva produced by the salivary glands lubricates the food and contains *amylase* enzymes that begin the digestion of starches. The chewed food or *chyme* now passes down the esophagus and enters the stomach. In the stomach, the chyme is further broken down by highly acidic gastric juice produced by the stomach lining. The enzyme *pepsin* is released by cells in the stomach lining to begin digestion of proteins. Muscular contractions of the stomach wall also serve to further grind the chyme into a smooth liquid. The chyme is now driven into the small intestine by contraction of the stomach. In the small intestine, further digestion of proteins, sugars and nucleotides/nucleosides will occur via intestinal and pancreatic enzymes. The small intestine is also where the majority of nutrient absorption occurs. By the time the remaining chyme has reached the large intestine, most of the available nutrients have been absorbed from it. The large intestine functions mainly in the absorption of water as well as the synthesis of vitamin K and certain B vitamins.

Disorders of the G.I. tract may be localized to a particular structure or organ or may be generalized throughout. Most G.I. disorders share some common symptoms that are listed in Table 16.1.

Table 16.1 General Symptoms of G.I. Disease

Anorexia — loss of appetite
Nausea
Vomiting
Diarrhea, constipation
Bleeding — obvious or "occult" (i.e., detected by laboratory test)

Abnormalities of the esophagus

Dysphagia

- Difficulty swallowing that may be caused by obstruction of the esophagus or impaired motility of the esophageal walls.
- Obstruction may be caused by tumors, congenital narrowing or diverticula (see below).
- Neurologic disorders such as brain injury, stroke or Parkinson's disease may affect voluntary swallowing or peristalsis of the esophagus.

Achalasia

- A condition caused by failure of the lower esophageal sphincter (cardiac sphincter) to relax and allow food to enter the stomach. It may be related to defects in neural input to the esophagus.
- Achalasia is a chronic condition that causes distention of the lower esophagus that may lead to chronic inflammation and eventual ulceration of the esophagus.
- The condition presents with dysphagia, vomiting and chest pain that is often exacerbated by eating.
- Aspiration of esophageal contents into the lungs is possible when lying down.

Esophageal diverticulum

- Diverticula are outpocketings of the esophageal walls that occur most frequently from congenital weakness of the esophagus walls.
- Food can easily become trapped in these diverticula, leading to inflammation and infection of the esophagus with possible ulceration.

Gastroesophageal reflux disease

- Gastroesophageal reflux is a condition caused by the backflow of stomach contents into the esophagus.
- It results from weakness or incompetence of the lower esophageal sphincter that normally blocks reflux of stomach contents into the esophagus.
- Because of their high acid content (low pH), reflux of stomach contents will cause irritation and inflammation of the esophagus (*esophagitis*) that can lead to ulceration of the esophagus.
- A *hiatal hernia* may also cause gastroesophageal reflux. A hiatal hernia is a protrusion of the top of the stomach through the opening of the diaphragm.

Manifestations

- Burning pain in the epigastric region ("heartburn") that may be worsened by alcohol consumption, caffeine, smoking, exercise and obesity. Reflux may also be worsened by lying down.
- Esophagitis, possible ulceration of esophagus.
- Dysphagia, poor nutrition.
- Possible increased risk of esophageal cancer with chronic esophagitis.

Table 16.2 Drugs for Treatment of Peptic Ulcer Disease

Antibiotics for eradication of *H. pylori* if present
Antacids (Examples: *magnesium hydroxide, aluminum hydroxide*)
Act by neutralizing gastric acid and raising gastric pH
Possible unwanted effects may include diarrhea or constipation
H_2 receptor antagonists (examples: *Ranitidine, Cimetidine*)
Inhibit the action of histamine at H_2 receptors to inhibit gastric acid secretion
Unwanted effects may include diarrhea, muscle pain and rashes
Proton-pump inhibitors (example: *Omeprazole*)
Block the intestinal H^+/K^+-ATPase pump to inhibit gastric acid secretion
Unwanted effects may include headache, diarrhea and rashes
Mucosal protective agents (examples: *bismuth, sucralfate*)
Enhance the mucosal protective barriers or provide an additional physical barrier over the surface of the G.I. tract
Unwanted effects are few but may include constipation

Treatment

- Consumption of frequent small meals rather than large ones.
- Sleeping with head elevated.
- Consumption of fluids with meals to wash food out of the esophagus.
- Use of antacids or proton pump inhibitors (see Table 16.2) to reduce pH of stomach contents.
- Surgery if a hiatal hernia is present.

Disorders of the stomach

Gastritis

- Gastritis refers to inflammation of the gastric mucosa (stomach lining).
- It may present as an acute or chronic disorder.

Acute gastritis

- Transient irritation and inflammation of the stomach lining.
- May be caused by factors such as alcohol consumption, aspirin use and stress.
- The inflammation associated with acute gastritis is a self-limiting process that does not usually result in long-term injury to the gastric mucosa.

Chronic gastritis

- Chronic irritation and inflammation of the stomach lining.

- May be caused by bacterial infection, alcohol abuse or long-term aspirin and nonsteroidal anti-inflammatory drug (NSAID) use.
- Can lead to atrophy and ulceration of the gastric mucosa.

Peptic ulcers

The term *peptic ulcer* refers to erosion of the mucosa lining any portion of the G.I. tract. If the ulcer occurs in the stomach lining, it is specifically referred to as a *gastric ulcer.* In the United States most ulcers occur in the duodenum and in elderly patients. The causes of peptic ulcer disease include the following:

- Infection with the bacteria *Helicobacter pylori* occurs in 80 to 95% of patients with peptic ulcer disease. *H. pylori* infection impairs the protective mechanisms of the G.I. tract against low pH and digestive enzymes and leads to ulceration of the mucosa.
- Stress — Emotional, trauma, surgical.
- Injury or death of mucus-producing cells.
- Excess acid production in the stomach. The hormone *gastrin* stimulates the production of acid in the stomach; therefore, any factors that increase gastrin production will in turn increase the production of stomach acid (see *Zollinger–Ellison syndrome* box).
- Chronic use of aspirins and NSAIDs.

Zollinger–Ellison syndrome

- Tumors of the gastrin-secreting endocrine cells of the pancreas or, less frequently, the duodenal wall.
- Leads to excessive acid production by the G.I. tract.
- Development of serious and aggressive peptic ulcers.
- Formation of ulcers in atypical locations.
- Complications can include perforation, hemorrhage and obstruction.
- Treatment may include resection of tumor, administration of H_2 receptor antagonists, anticholinergics and antacids.

Manifestations of peptic ulcer disease

- Episodes of remission and exacerbation
- Pain that for duodenal ulcers is often relieved by eating or antacids
- G.I. bleeding and possible hemorrhage (20 to 25% of patients)
- Perforation of ulcers with significant mortality
- Obstruction of G.I. tract

Treatment of peptic ulcer disease

- Avoidance of alcohol, smoking and NSAIDs
- Antibiotic therapy, which has been shown to be highly effective in eradicating *H. pylori* in the vast majority of patients (see Table 16.2)
- Antacids
- H_2 antagonists
- Mucosal protectants

Disorders of the intestines

Irritable bowel syndrome

- May be one of the most common G.I. disorders.
- Patients present with symptoms of G.I. pain, gas, bloating and altered bowel function (diarrhea or constipation). Most symptoms are localized to the lower intestine and colon.
- No underlying pathophysiologic processes have yet to be identified in these patients. "Hyperreactivity" and excessive motility of the bowels may be contributing factors.
- Emotional factors and diet may exacerbate the symptoms.
- Treatment may include psychological counseling, dietary changes such as increased fiber consumption. Antidiarrhea, anticholinergic and antispasmodic agents might also be of value.

Inflammatory bowel disease

The term *inflammatory bowel disease* includes the conditions *Crohn's disease* and *ulcerative colitis*. Both of these diseases are characterized by chronic inflammation of various regions of the G.I. tract (see Table 16.3).

Table 16.3 Comparison of Key Characteristics in Crohn's Disease and Ulcerative Colitis

	Crohn's disease	Ulcerative colitis
Age of onset	10–40 years	10–30 years
Location	Large intestine	Large or small intestine
Inflammation	"Skip" lesions	Uniform and continuous
Layers involved	Mainly submucosal	Mainly mucosal
Bloody stool	Rare	Common
Diarrhea	Common	Common
Malabsorption	Rare	Common
Cancer risk	Increased	Unchanged?
Abdominal pain	Mild to severe	Mild to severe

Crohn's disease

- Although the exact etiology of Crohn's disease in unknown, there appears to be a significant autoimmune component. Much recent interest has focused on the possible role of pro-inflammatory *cytokines* in the pathogenesis of this disorder.
- The disease may affect any region of the G.I. tract but is most commonly seen in the distal ileum and colon.
- Distribution of Crohn's disease shows a distinct predisposition to certain populations including Jews and individuals from the United States, Western Europe and Scandinavia. The disease often presents in the late teens to early 20s and is present for the life of the patient with intermittent periods of remission and exacerbation.
- The inflammation of Crohn's disease is particularly evident in the *submucosal* layer of the intestine. The pattern of inflammation seen is a *granulomatous inflammation* with distinct "cobblestone" appearance to the mucosa. The inflammatory lesions are not constant along the length of the intestine but rather present with a "skip" pattern that intersperses areas of inflammation with normal looking, non-inflamed tissue.

Manifestations of Crohn's disease

- Diarrhea (blood is usually not evident in the stool but may be occult, i.e., detected by clinical assay)
- Intestinal pain similar to indigestion
- Fever
- Weight loss from intestinal malabsorption
- Nausea, anorexia, vomiting
- Complications: intestinal obstruction, formation of *fistulas* (abnormal connections between the colon and other abdominal organs)
- Toxic megacolon

Toxic megacolon

- Life-threatening distention of the colon.
- May lead to perforation of the colon, septicemia and peritonitis.
- Mortality associated with a perforated colon is on the order of 40% or more.

Treatment of Crohn's disease

- Nutritional supplementation to offset the poor nutrition that can result from anorexia and intestinal malabsorption. Total parenteral nutrition may be indicated in severe cases.
- Anti-inflammatory drugs.
- Recently, considerable research has focused on the role of pro-inflammatory cytokines in Crohn's disease and the possibility that drugs or antibodies that block cytokine action might be of benefit in treating the disease.

Ulcerative colitis

- Inflammatory disease of the rectum and colon.
- The disease primarily affects the *submucosa* layer of the intestines.
- Unlike Crohn's disease the pattern of inflammation is continuous throughout the affected area.
- Like Crohn's disease, ulcerative colitis also presents with periods of remission and exacerbation.
- Although the exact etiology of ulcerative colitis is unknown, genetic and immunological factors are likely contributors to the disease. Individuals between the ages of 20 and 40 are most susceptible, particularly those with a family history of the disorder or who are of Jewish descent.

Manifestations of ulcerative colitis

- Chronic, bloody diarrhea
- Fever, pain
- Weight loss
- Possible anemia from blood loss
- Possible complications: *toxic megacolon*, perforation of the intestine, significant blood loss; an increased incidence of colon cancer has also been documented in patients with ulcerative colitis

Treatment of ulcerative colitis

- Anti-inflammatory drugs and salicylates suppress the inflammatory response.
- Sulfasalazine — A combination sulfa and aminosalicylate drug.
- Nicotine appears to exert a protective effect in ulcerative colitis but not Crohn's disease.
- Severe malnutrition may require nutritional supplementation.
- Surgical resection of diseased bowel may be required.

Disorders of the gall bladder

The gall bladder is a saclike structure that stores the bile that is produced by the liver. The walls of the gall bladder contain smooth muscle and, under the stimulus of the duodenal hormone *cholecystokinin*, can contract to eject bile down the bile duct and into the duodenum. In the duodenum, bile salts emulsify fats to aid in their absorption. Bile is composed primarily of water, bile salts, cholesterol and bilirubin.

Gallstone formation (cholelithiasis)

- Cholelithiasis is the most common disorder of the G.I. system.
- The gallstones that form in the gall bladder are hardened precipitates of bile that contain predominantly cholesterol.
- The size of gallstones can range from the size of a grain of sand to several inches in diameter.
- Factors such as aging, excess cholesterol, obesity, sudden dietary changes or abnormal fat metabolism may contribute to gallstone formation.
- Gallstones may be detected by a number of techniques including radiography, ultrasonography and cholecystoscopy.

Manifestations of gallstone formation

- Symptoms of gallstone formation will generally not occur until the stones have reached sufficient size to block the bile ducts.
- Acute and severe abdominal pain.
- Nausea, vomiting, fever, chills.
- Jaundice from obstruction of bile outflow.

Treatment

- Surgical removal of gall bladder (*cholecystectomy*)
- Endoscopic removal of gallstones
- *Lithotripsy* — The use of sound waves to break up the gallstones in the gall bladder
- Low-fat diet for prevention of additional stone formation

Cholecystitis

Cholecystitis is an acute or chronic inflammation of the gall bladder. It is most commonly caused by the presence of gallstones in the gall bladder, but may also result from infection or reduced blood flow to the gall bladder. Signs and symptoms are similar to those observed with cholelithiasis. Treatment involves removal of gallstones and antibiotics for treatment of infection if present.

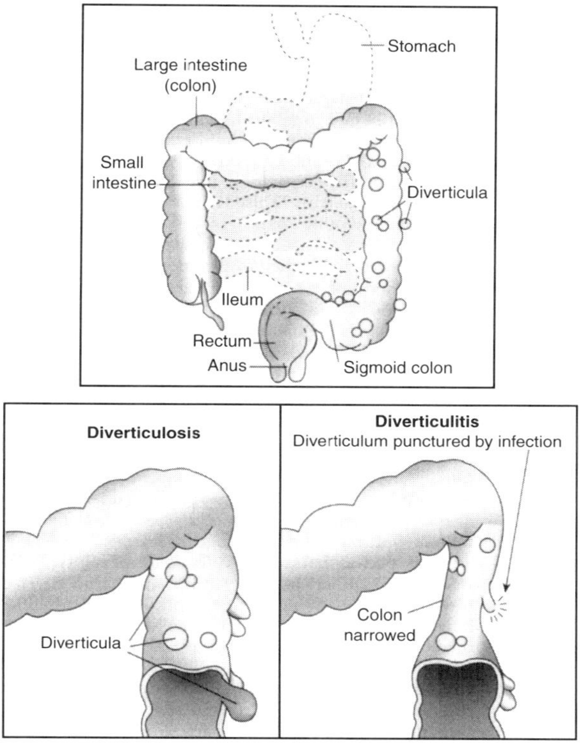

Figure 16.1 Diverticulum in colon (top). Diverticulosis (bottom left). Diverticulitis (bottom right). (From Porth, C.M., *Pathophysiology: Concepts of Altered Health States*, 5th ed., Lippincott, Philadelphia, 1998. With permission.)

Diverticular disease

Diverticular disease is a condition characterized by the presence of *diverticula*, which are multiple saclike protrusions of the mucosa. *True diverticula* involve all layers of the intestinal wall, whereas *false diverticula* involve only the muscularis. Diverticular disease occurs with increased frequency in elderly individuals and may be associated with age-related changes in the bowel. Individuals who consume a low-fiber, low-bulk diet also appear at greater risk for the formation of diverticula (see Figure 16.1).

Manifestations of diverticular disease

- Often asymptomatic
- Changes in bowel habits
- Excess flatulence
- A possible serious complication of diverticular disease is infection or inflammation of the diverticula (*diverticulitis*) due to trapping of intes-

tinal contents and accumulation of intestinal contents in the diverticula. This may lead to eventual perforation of the intestinal wall and sepsis.

Treatment of diverticular disease

- Increased bulk and fiber in the diet
- Antibiotics if diverticulitis is present

Colorectal cancer

Colorectal cancer is the second leading cause of cancer deaths in the United States after lung cancer. Most cases of colorectal cancer are carcinomas that arise from preexisting colorectal *polyps*. A number of factors may contribute to the development of colorectal cancer, including high-fat diet, low-fiber diet, age over 50 years and genetic predisposition. Colorectal cancer may be detected though proctoscopy, by the presence of occult blood in the stool or by blood tests for the presence of several tumor-specific antigens.

Definition

Polyp — A mass of tissue that projects outward or upward from the bowel wall and protrudes into the lumen.

Manifestations of colorectal cancer

- Diarrhea or constipation
- Blood in the stool (obvious or occult)
- Rarely pain
- Weakness, malaise, anorexia, weight loss
- Bowel obstruction
- Common sites of metastasis for colorectal cancer: the brain, lungs and bone
- Long-term prognosis dependent on how early the cancer is detected and the extent to which it has spread

chapter seventeen

Disease of the liver and exocrine pancreas

Study objectives

- List the major functions of the liver.
- Discuss the key features of the hepatitis A to E viruses in terms of their epidemiology, effects on the liver and possible long-term consequences.
- Define cirrhosis.
- Describe the three stages of alcoholic liver disease.
- List the major manifestations of cirrhosis. Why does each of these manifestations occur?
- What are interferons? Discuss their usefulness in viral hepatitis.
- Define jaundice. Why might it occur?
- Discuss acute and chronic pancreatitis. What might cause each? What are some of the possible effects of each on the body?

Introduction

The liver is a large glandular organ comprising two main lobes. The large left and right lobes of the human liver are further subdivided into a number of smaller lobules. The liver is responsible for performing a number of crucial functions that are essential for normal life (see Table 17.1). Alteration of liver function may result from exposure to a number of factors such as viruses, alcohol, toxins and drugs and can result in conditions such as *hepatitis* and *cirrhosis*. In light of the many key functions of the liver, factors that affect liver function will often have profound effects on normal physiology and function.

Table 17.1 Functions of the Liver

Functions of the Liver
Carbohydrate, fat and protein metabolism
Metabolism of steroid and sex hormones
Production of bile
Elimination of bilirubin
Drug metabolism
Synthesis of plasma proteins and clotting factors
Storage of glycogen, minerals and vitamins

Viral hepatitis

The term *hepatitis* refers to inflammation and possible injury of the liver. Hepatitis may be caused by a number of injurious agents such as viruses, alcohol, toxins and drugs. When the liver is inflamed and injured as a result of viral infection it is termed a *viral hepatitis*. Alcoholic hepatitis will be discussed under the topic of cirrhosis. In the United States, there are three main hepatitis viruses, designated hepatitis A, B and C. Two other variants, hepatitis D and E are also present in certain populations. All of the hepatitis viruses target the hepatocytes of the liver as their site of infection and replication. Because many of the clinical features of the various hepatitis viruses are quite similar, the manifestations of hepatitis infection will be discussed as a group (see Table 17.2).

Table 17.2 Characteristics of Viral Hepatitis

	Hepatitis virus				
	A	B	C	D	E
Incubation (days)	15–50	30–180	15–160	30–180	10–60
Transmission	F/O	BBF	BBF	BBF	F/O
Onset	Abrupt	Insidious	Insidious	Insidious	Abrupt
Chronic hepatitis	Rare	Possible	Possible	Possible	Unlikely

F/O = fecal/oral; BBF = blood and body fluids.

Epidemiology

1. Hepatitis A
   - Transmitted via the fecal/oral route, usually through fecal-contaminated food, water or shellfish. Numerous outbreaks have been traced to infected food handlers. The highest incidence occurs in children and adolescents, and in the United States outbreaks are sometimes seen in day-care centers.
   - The virus may also be transmitted via blood and contaminated blood products but this is not the primary means of transmission.
2. Hepatitis B
   - Blood-borne pathogen.
   - Major routes of transmission include intravenous drug use, unprotected sexual contact (heterosexual and homosexual) and exposure to contaminated blood products.
3. Hepatitis C
   - Blood-borne pathogen.
   - Major route of transmission is through contaminated blood and body fluids.
   - Accounts for most cases of transfusion-related viral hepatitis.
4. Hepatitis D
   - Blood-borne pathogen.
   - Can only infect individuals with active hepatitis B infection.
   - Transmitted through contaminated blood and body fluids.
5. Hepatitis E
   - Fecal/oral route of transmission.
   - Outbreaks are more common in developing nations and refugee camps due to poor sanitation and fecal contamination of water supplies.
   - Young children are most frequently affected.
   - The effects of hepatitis E infection are particularly severe in pregnant women.

Manifestations of viral hepatitis

- Range from asymptomatic to severe
- Fatigue, malaise, anorexia, nausea
- *Jaundice* (see box and Figure 17.1)
- Liver inflammation and abdominal pain
- Abnormal liver function and enzyme levels

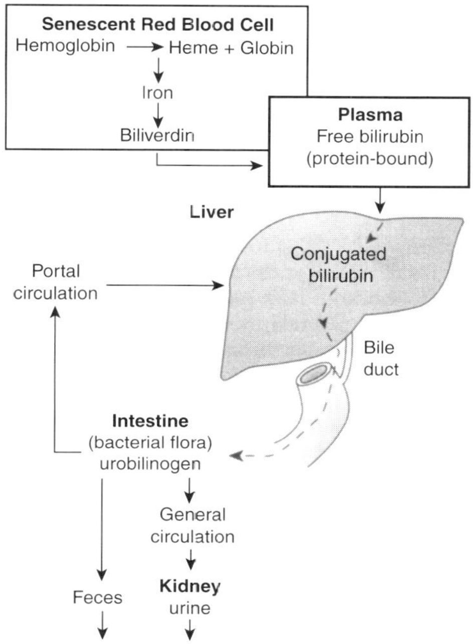

Figure 17.1 Bilirubin formation and elimination. (From Porth, C.M., *Pathophysiology: Concepts of Altered Health States*, 5th ed., Lippincott, Philadelphia, 1998. With permission.)

Jaundice

A yellowing of the skin and whites of the eyes due to excess levels of circulating bilirubin. Bilirubin is formed from hemoglobin during the normal and abnormal breakdown of red blood cells. Free bilirubin formed in the blood is conjugated by the liver and eliminated into the intestinal tract along with bile. Any condition that impairs the ability of the liver to conjugate and eliminate bilirubin will result in the accumulation of bilirubin in the blood with accompanying jaundice.

Possible complications of hepatitis

- Chronic active or persistent hepatitis can lead to progressive liver injury, liver failure and death. The chronic form of hepatitis is most common with hepatitis B, C, D, but rare with hepatitis A and E.
- Chronic active hepatitis is also associated with an increased incidence of hepatocellular carcinoma.

Treatment of hepatitis

- Many hepatitis infections will resolve within 4 to 8 weeks without treatment. Hepatitis A rarely becomes chronic and seldom requires treatment other than supportive measures. The long-term course of hepatitis B and C is less predictable.
- Therapies for chronic hepatitis are currently few and their effectiveness is quite variable. *Alpha interferon* is currently approved for treatment of chronic hepatitis B and C in the United States (see Interferons box). Biochemical and histologic improvement is seen in approximately 25 to 50% of patients with hepatitis B treated with alpha interferon.[19]
- Effective vaccines are currently available against hepatitis A, B and C.

Interferons

- A group of endogenous cytokines that possess antiviral and immunomodulating properties.
- The antiviral effects of the interferons appear to be mediated through a number of mechanisms including inhibition of viral penetration, uncoating and synthesis of viral proteins.
- Interferons must be administered though intramuscular or subcutaneous injection.
- Interferon alpha is currently most promising in treating chronic hepatitis.
- Side effects of interferon therapy can include flulike symptoms. Dose-limiting toxicities of interferon use are blood cell toxicity and neurotoxicity.

Cirrhosis

Cirrhosis is a general term referring to destruction of normal liver structure. Cirrhosis is characterized by diffuse scarring and fibrosis of the liver in response to chronic inflammation and injury. One of the major features of cirrhosis is the replacement of functional liver tissue by scar tissue. The most prevalent cause of liver cirrhosis is alcohol abuse (see Table 17.3). Alcoholic liver disease presents in three progressive stages.

Stages of alcoholic liver disease

- Alcoholic steatosis — "Fatty liver." Accumulation of fat in the hepatocytes. May occur as a result of altered fat metabolism in the liver. Changes include increased synthesis of fatty acids and triglycerides.

Table 17.3 Cirrhosis of the Liver

Alcoholic cirrhosis (portal cirrhosis, Laennec cirrhosis) — Caused by excess ethanol intake, and possible acetaldehyde toxicity (a metabolite of ethanol)
Biliary cirrhosis — Caused by bile duct obstruction (intrahepatic or extrahepatic)
Post-necrotic cirrhosis - Caused by viral hepatitis, exposure to drugs or toxins
Metabolic Cirrhosis — caused by Glycogen Storage Disease, Wilson disease, α-1-antitrypsin deficiency, galactosemia

Enlargement of the liver is accompanied by symptoms that may include anorexia, nausea and jaundice. At this point the fatty changes are generally reversible if alcohol consumption ceases.

- Alcoholic hepatitis — Inflammation, degeneration and necrosis of hepatocytes with continued alcohol intake. Symptoms can range from mild to severe and can include anorexia and weight loss. Structural changes in alcoholic hepatitis are also reversible to a large extent if alcohol consumption ceases.
- Alcoholic cirrhosis — Diffuse scarring and fibrosis of the liver that occurs after many years of alcohol abuse. Because the liver plays such an important role in many normal physiologic processes, alcoholic cirrhosis is a multisystem disease.

Manifestations of alcoholic cirrhosis

- Hepatosplenomegaly
- *Ascites* — Accumulation of fluid in the peritoneal cavity; results from portal hypertension and decreased plasma protein production by the liver; presents with massive distention of the abdomen
- *Portal hypertension* (see box)
- *Hepatorenal syndrome* — Renal failure that can accompany advanced liver disease
- Edema
- Jaundice
- Hepatic encephalopathy — Neurologic dysfunction that can accompany advanced liver disease; may be caused in part by the accumulation of ammonia and other toxins in the circulation
- Distention of abdominal and esophageal veins (*esophageal varices*) due to increased portal and venous pressures; *caput medusae* is a term used to describe the distended abdominal veins that are seen in patients with alcoholic cirrhosis
- Reduced metabolism of circulating sex hormones can result in gynecomastia, menstrual irregularities, abnormal sexual function
- Liver failure

Portal hypertension

- Elevated portal blood pressure caused by increased resistance to blood flow through the liver as a result of scar tissue.
- The increased portal pressure causes the backing up of blood into the spleen (splenomegaly) as well as collateral blood vessels of the abdomen and esophagus causing varices.
- Symptoms include bleeding of varices, ascites and splenomegaly with possible destruction of platelets and other blood cells.

Treatment of cirrhosis

- Nutritional and vitamin supplementation. A reduced-protein diet is useful to decrease ammonia production.
- Diuretics to relieve fluid accumulation.
- Intubation or shunting to relieve bleeding from accessory blood vessels.
- Management of symptoms of liver failure.

Liver cancer

Tumors originating in the liver are rare but tend to be malignant when they arise and are usually symptomatic. More commonly, tumors arise outside of the liver and spread to it as a result of metastasis. Because of its rich blood supply, the liver provides an excellent site for growth of metastatic tumors. Lung, breast, colon and pancreatic tumors are the most common source of metastatic tumors to the liver. The clinical manifestations of liver cancer or metastasis will depend primarily on the rate of tumor growth. As more functional liver tissue becomes involved, the clinical manifestations tend to become more severe. Growing tumors may impair liver blood flow and bile outflow, leading to hepatomegaly and jaundice. *Cachexia* or lean tissue wasting tends to be severe with liver cancer or metastasis (see Chapter 2). Long-term prognosis is poor.

Disorders of the pancreas — Pancreatitis

Pancreatitis is inflammation of the pancreas that may be acute or chronic. The possible causes of acute and chronic pancreatitis are listed in Table 17.4.

Manifestations

- Epigastric pain
- Fever, nausea, vomiting

Table 17.4 Pancreatitis

Acute
Many instances do not have a clear cause; may involve inflammation due to abnormal release of pancreatic enzymes or reflux of duodenal contents into pancreatic tissues
May also be caused by blockage of pancreatic outflow through the common bile duct by gallstones
May be caused in rare instances by certain drugs such as thiazide diuretics, NSAIDS or sulfonamide antibiotics
Infectious agents
Chronic
Alcohol abuse the most common cause of chronic pancreatitis
May also be caused by pancreatic tumors or cysts
May lead to irreversible changes in pancreas structure and function

- Reduced bowel activity
- Anorexia, malaise
- Intestinal malabsorption, poor digestion of nutrients
- Diabetes mellitus if endocrine function of the pancreas is compromised

Treatment

- Prevention of intestinal malabsorption
- Exogenous oral replacement of pancreatic enzymes
- Antibiotics for infection if present
- Pain medication
- Drugs to decrease gastric acid secretion
- Surgical drainage

chapter eighteen

Endocrine disorders

Study objectives

- Describe the anatomic and functional relationship between the hypothalamus and pituitary gland.
- List the various hormones of the anterior and posterior pituitary along with their main actions.
- Discuss the main differences between acromegaly and gigantism.
- Distinguish idiopathic short stature from familial short stature.
- Distinguish cretinism from myxedema. Why does each occur and how do they differ from one another?
- List the main symptoms of hyperthyroidism and hypothyroidism.
- Define toxic and nontoxic goiter.
- List the cause and key manifestations of each of the following disorders:
  Congenital adrenal hyperplasia
  Addison's disease
  Cushing's disease
- What is a pheochromocytoma? What effects does it have on the body?
- Define diabetes insipidus.

Introduction

Glands of the endocrine system secrete various hormones that play a key role in maintaining normal homeostasis as well allowing the body to deal with periods of physiologic stress. Abnormalities of endocrine glands generally fall into one of the several categories:

1. Hypersecretion
    - Excess activity of a specific hormone or hormones
    - May be due to overproduction of a hormone due to abnormal glandular function, glandular hypertrophy/hyperplasia or the presence of tumors that secrete hormone
2. Hyposecretion
    - Reduced activity of a specific hormone or hormones
    - May be due to atrophy of glandular tissue or damage from autoimmune attack, infection or neoplasia
3. Altered responsiveness of a tissue to a specific hormone
    - Tissue no longer responds to a specific hormone
    - May involve downregulation of receptors or altered receptor/secondary messenger function
    - Circulating levels of hormone may be normal or even elevated (example: type II diabetes)

Abnormalities of the hypothalamus/pituitary glands

The *hypothalamus* is often referred to as the "master gland" of the body by virtue of its regulatory role over other glands. The hypothalamus lies at the base of the brain and receives neural input from a number of higher brain regions. These neural connections allow the hypothalamus to integrate many of the interactions between the autonomic nervous system and endocrine system. The hypothalamus is connected to the *pituitary* gland through a stalk called the *infundibulum*. Hypothalamic releasing hormones are carried by a blood vessel portal system found within the infundibulum to the anterior pituitary where they in turn stimulate the release of specific hormones from the anterior pituitary. Two hormones of the posterior pituitary (oxytocin and vasopressin) are actually synthesized in neuron clusters within the hypothalamus and transported down axons to the posterior pituitary where they are released. A summary of the hypothalamic and pituitary hormones is given in Tables 18.1 and 18.2.

Injury to the hypothalamus can lead to a decreased production of hypothalamic hormones. In light of the many hormones released in response to hypothalamic releasing hormones, manifestations of abnormal hypothalamic function are numerous. Release of pituitary hormones (LH, FSH, GH, ACTH, etc.) is impaired as is release of thyroid hormones as a result of TRH deficiency.

Table 18.1 Hormones of the Hypothalamus

Growth hormone-releasing hormone (GHRH) — Stimulates the release of growth hormone (GH) from the anterior pituitary
Gonadotrophin-releasing hormone (GnRH) — Stimulates release of luteinizing hormone (LH) and follicle-stimulating hormone (FSH) from the anterior pituitary
Thryotrophin-releasing hormone (TRH) — Stimulates the release of thyroid-stimulating hormone (TSH) and prolactin (PRL) from the anterior pituitary
Corticotrophin-releasing hormone (CRH) — Stimulates the release of adrenocorticotrophin (ACTH) from the anterior pituitary
Somatostatin — Inhibits the release of growth hormone from the anterior pituitary

Table 18.2 Hormones of the Pituitary

Hormones of the anterior pituitary
- *Growth hormone* (GH) — Stimulates growth of long bones, organs and muscle during development
- *Adrenocorticotrophin* (ACTH) — Stimulates the adrenal cortex to produce adrenal hormones such as cortisol
- *Thyroid-stimulating hormone* (TSH) — Regulates secretion of thyroid hormones T_3 and T_4
- *Luteinizing hormone* (LH) — Stimulates steroidogenesis in the gonads, maintains secretory function of the corpus luteum
- *Follicle-stimulating hormone* (FSH) — Stimulates gamete production in the gonads
- *Prolactin* (PRL) — Initiates and maintains milk production in the mammary glands postpartum

Hormones of the posterior pituitary
- *Oxytocin* — Stimulates contraction of uterine smooth muscle during labor and delivery as well as milk ejection from the mammary glands
- *Antidiuretic hormone* (ADH, vasopressin) — Acts on the kidney to stimulate water reabsorption in the distal tubules and collecting ducts

Hypopituitarism

- Decreased activity of the pituitary gland along with hyposecretion of one or more pituitary hormones. If all pituitary hormones are lacking, it is termed *panhypopituitarism.*
- Most commonly results from damage to the pituitary (trauma, infection, ischemia or tumors).
- Manifestations are highly variable and depend on the hormone or hormones that are lacking. For the effects of specific hormone deficiency see the following sections.

Disorders of the anterior pituitary gland

Alterations of growth hormone secretion

Growth hormone is a polypeptide that is synthesized and secreted by the anterior pituitary gland. Growth hormone stimulates the growth of cartilage, long bones, muscle and organs during childhood development.

Growth hormone hyposecretion

- In children and adolescents, GH secretion occurs in a pulsatile fashion at night and during sleep. Daytime levels of GH are very low and not indicative of overall GH release. To evaluate GH secretion in a particular patient it is important to take samples throughout a 24-hour period.
- Deficiency of GH secretion may occur from a congenital defect in the pituitary gland or may be acquired as a result of injury or tumor growth. Growth hormone deficiency is also seen in congenital conditions such as Turner syndrome and Down syndrome. Many cases of GH deficiency are *idiopathic,* meaning their cause cannot be clearly identified.

Manifestations

- The major manifestation of growth hormone deficiency in children is short stature.
- Delayed development of muscle and bone may also occur.

Growth hormone, the fountain of youth?

Growth hormone secretion decreases as we age. There is a significant body of evidence that this drop in growth hormone secretion contributes to the loss of muscle and skin tone that we experience as we age. A number of studies in reputable journals have reported that supplemental growth hormone administration can slow and even reverse some of the undesirable effects of aging on the body.[20] In certain countries, there are "spas" that include growth hormone replacement therapy as part of their youth-restoring regimens. However, long-term growth hormone replacement therapy is very expensive and may be associated with the development of glucose intolerance, diabetes and even certain types of cancers. Does the risk outweigh the potential benefits?

Treatment

- Many patients with idiopathic growth hormone deficiency and resulting short stature will benefit from GH replacement therapy in terms of final height and development.
- The use of GH supplementation in children with *familial short stature* (children who are normal but who will be short because their parents were short) is controversial. Although these children might experience some modest increase in final height, GH replacement therapy is very expensive and may be associated with an increased risk of diabetes and leukemia.

Growth hormone hypersecretion — Gigantism and acromegaly

- Gigantism results from the excess production of growth hormone before the epiphyseal growth plates of the long bones fuse (around puberty).
- Acromegaly is growth hormone excess that occurs after the epiphyseal growth plates of the long bones fuse.
- Both conditions are most commonly caused by a tumor of the anterior pituitary gland.

Manifestations

- Extremely tall stature with gigantism due to excessive growth of the long bones.
- Overgrowth of connective tissues with acromegaly. Although bones can no longer grow in length, they can grow in thickness. Patients present with thickening and deformation of the hands, face, skull and feet.
- Patients also tend to have very oily skin.
- Central nervous system disturbances (headache, vision changes) and abnormalities may occur.
- Cardiovascular disease in the form of hypertension and coronary artery disease represents a significant source of mortality in these patients.

Treatment

- Surgical removal of tumor. Note that secretion of other pituitary hormones may be altered as a result of tumor removal.
- Radiation therapy of the tumor may be performed if surgery is not feasible.

Disorders of the posterior pituitary

Syndrome of inappropriate ADH (SIADH)

- A condition characterized by excess production of ADH from the posterior pituitary.
- May be caused by pituitary tumors or injury. Can also occur transiently due to physiologic stress.

Manifestations

- Excessive water retention
- Weight gain due to water accumulation
- Alterations in serum sodium levels

Treatment

- Fluid restriction
- Diuretics
- Removal of tumor if present

Diabetes insipidus

- A condition caused by decreased production of ADH.
- May result from defects in the hypothalamus/pituitary or from a tumor or trauma.
- A *nephrogenic* form of diabetes insipidus also occurs in which ADH production is normal but the kidneys do not respond to the effects of ADH.

Manifestations

- Production of excessive amounts of very dilute urine
- Increased plasma osmolarity
- Possible hypotension and reflex tachycardia
- Possible dehydration and excessive thirst (*polydyspsia*)

Treatment

Administration of ADH and ADH analogues like *lypressin* (Lys^8-vasopressin) and *desmopressin* (1-deamino-D-Arg^8-vasopressin). ADH itself is administered by subcutaneous or intramuscular injection, whereas lypressin and desmopressin are administered as an intranasal spray. An oral form of desmopressin is also now available. ADH replacement is generally lifelong.

Alteration of thyroid function

There are two main hormones produced by the thyroid gland: *thyroxin* (T_4) and *triiodothyronine* (T_3). Both hormones are derived from the amino acid *tyrosine* and contain *iodine* that is extracted from the blood. The release of thyroid hormones from the anterior pituitary is regulated by TRH secreted from the anterior pituitary gland. The main actions of T_3 and T_4 are outlined in Table 18.3.

Hypothyroidism

- May be a primary condition resulting from a defect within the thyroid itself or can be secondary to a lack of stimulation by TSH.
- Dietary deficiency of *iodine* may lead to hypertrophy of the thyroid gland that presents as a *goiter* (see Table 18.4).
- The most common cause of hypothyroidism is an autoimmune condition called *Hashimoto's thyroiditis* in which antibodies are produced against the tissue of the thyroid. Although the exact etiology of this autoimmune disorder is unknown, it can lead to progressive destruction of the thyroid gland and loss of thyroid function.

Manifestations

Cretinism

- Hypothyroidism that occurs during fetal development
- May occur as a result of a congenital defect in thyroid development
- Severe mental retardation due to poor development of the brain
- Poor overall development and growth retardation

Table 18.3 Physiologic Effects of Thyroid Hormones

Increased basal metabolic rate
Maintenance of normal metabolic function
Development of the nervous system in the fetus

Table 18.4 Toxic Goiter and Nontoxic Goiter

Nontoxic goiter — Hypertrophy of the thyroid gland that is not accompanied by excess secretion of thyroid hormones. May occur as a result of dietary iodine deficiency. Symptoms are those of hypothyroidism.
Toxic goiter — Hypertrophy of the thyroid that is accompanied by excess thyroid production. May be associated with *Grave's disease*. Symptoms are those of hyperthyroidism. *Thyrotoxicosis* is a term that is used to describe the "toxic" effects of excess thyroid hormones on the body.

Myxedema

- Hypothyroidism in the adult
- May result from autoimmune destruction of the thyroid or thyroid injury or removal
- Presents with signs of hypometabolism including:
  Cold intolerance
  Weight gain
  Fatigue
  Bradycardia
  Cool, dry skin
  Anorexia
  Constipation
  Edema of the face (swelling around the eyes), hands and ankles; drooping eyelids
- Possible long-term complications of untreated hypothyroidism, including cardiac hypertrophy, heart failure, and *myxedema coma,* which presents with hypothermia, seizures and respiratory depression

Treatment

Thyroid hormone replacement therapy. A variety of synthetic and natural T_3/T_4 preparations are available for use orally.

Hyperthyroidism

Increased synthesis and release of T_3 and T_4. Hyperthyroidism may be a primary condition that results from an overactive thyroid gland or it may occur as a result of excessive stimulation of the thyroid by TSH from the pituitary. Hyperthyroidism is also referred to as *thyrotoxicosis*. One of the most common causes of hyperthyroidism is *Grave's disease.* Hyperthyroidism can also be caused by a toxic goiter not associated with Grave's disease (*Plummer's disease*) or by a tumor of the thyroid. In rare cases carcinomas arising outside of the thyroid may produce thyroid hormone or TSH.

Grave's disease

Patients with Grave's disease produce antibodies that bind TSH receptors on the thyroid and mimic the actions of TSH leading to excess production of thyroid hormones.

Manifestations

The manifestations of hyperthyroidism are essentially the same regardless of the cause of the hyperthyroidism; they include the following:

- Increased basal metabolic rate
- Increased heat production, patient always feels "hot"

- Tachycardia
- Increased catecholamine sensitivity; patients are at risk for cardiac arrhythmias
- Increased appetite
- Weight loss
- Enhanced bowel activity
- Behavioral changes including possible nervousness and hyperactivity

Treatment

- β-Blocking drugs to blunt the effects of excess adrenergic stimulation.
- Antithyroid drugs (*propylthiouracil, carbimazole, methimazole*) that block production of thyroid hormone.
- *Radioiodine* — Given orally and taken up by hormone-producing cells of the thyroid as if it were normal iodine. The cytotoxic actions of the β and γ radiation destroy the hormone-producing cells of the thyroid. After treatment the patient usually becomes hypothyroid and must be managed with thyroid hormone replacement therapy. Radioactive iodine should not be used in patients of childbearing age due to the possible effects on offspring.
- Surgical ablation of a portion of the thyroid may also be used. Following surgery, patients may likewise become hypothyroid and require thyroid hormone replacement therapy.

Disorders of the adrenal glands

The adrenal glands are small, triangular structures that lie on top of the kidneys. Anatomically, the adrenal glands may be divided into two parts, the *adrenal medulla* and the *adrenal cortex*. The adrenal medulla contains cells that secrete the *catecholamines* epinephrine and norepinephrine. Cells of the adrenal cortex secrete the *glucocorticoids* (mainly *cortisol*), the *mineralcorticoids* (mainly *aldosterone*) and some *testosterone*. The physiologic functions of the adrenal hormones are shown in Table 18.5.

Hyposecretion of adrenal hormones

Congenital adrenal hypoplasia (CAH)

- An autosomal recessive disorder in which the enzymes necessary for cortisol synthesis are deficient.
- Lack of cortisol-negative feedback on the pituitary gland leads to excess ACTH production, which in turn increases the synthesis and release of androgens from the adenal cortex.
- Aldosterone production may also be altered depending on the specific enzyme(s) lacking.

Table 18.5 Physiologic Effects of Adrenal Hormones

Adrenal medulla
Catecholamines: Epinephrine and norepinephrine
Involved in the "fight or flight response"
Interact with α and β receptors in the body
Increase heart and respiratory rate
Increase energy availability; stimulate glycogenolysis in the liver as well as plasma levels of free fatty acids
Reduce gastrointestinal activity
Adrenal cortex
Glucocorticoids: Cortisol, corticosterone, cortisol
Stimulate the synthesis and storage of glycogen
Increase gluconeogenesis and blood glucose levels
Exert catabolic effects in muscle and fat tissue
Anti-inflammatory action; used clinically as anti-inflammatory agents
Mineralcorticoids: Aldosterone
Act on the distal tubules and collecting ducts of the kidney to increase reabsorption of sodium
Increase plasma volume
Increase renal excretion of potassium and protons

Manifestations

- Masculinization of the female external genitals (*pseudohemaphroditism*).
- Short stature due to premature fusion of the epiphyseal growth plate in the long bones.
- With certain forms of CAH, a lack of aldosterone production may lead to significant "salt wasting" (sodium losses).

Treatment

- Administration of cortisone/hydrocortisone will reduce ACTH levels and block the subsequent production of excess androgens.
- Serum electrolyte levels should be closely monitored and corrected, particularly in the salt-wasting form of CAH.
- Reconstructive surgery of the genitals may be necessary in females to alter the obvious male characteristics.

Addison's disease

- A primary condition associated with atrophy of the adrenal glands.
- The majority of cases arise from autoimmune destruction of the adrenal glands. Some cases may occur as a result of adrenal gland injury as a result of infection or tumors.

- Decreased production of cortisol, aldosterone and androgens from the adrenal glands.
- Decreased levels of glucocorticoids (cortisol) results in increased levels of ACTH.

Manifestations

- The manifestations of Addison's disease are due to deficiency of all three hormone groups produced by the adrenal gland (glucocorticoids, mineralcorticoids and androgens).
- Weakness and fatigue.
- Increased pigmentation of the skin due to an ACTH-induced increase in *melanocyte* (skin pigment cell) activity.
- Weight loss, anorexia, hypometabolism, cold intolerance.
- Cardiovascular changes — Hypotension, orthostatic hypotension, electrocardiographic changes.
- Changes in electroencephalogram and mental function.
- Although androgen production from the adrenal glands is reduced, androgen production from other sites in the body (testis) is sufficient to maintain normal sexual function and development.

Adrenal crisis

An episode of severe hypotension, vascular collapse, acute renal failure and hypothermia caused by a combined lack of cortisol and aldosterone. It may be precipitated by infection, trauma and dehydration in individuals with Addison's disease and can be life-threatening.

Treatment

- Lifelong replacement therapy with glucocorticoids (cortisone/hydrocortisone) and mineralcorticoids (aldosterone).

Cushing's disease

- Characterized by excess circulating levels of cortisol.
- May be caused by excess ACTH secretion due to pituitary tumors or a tumor of the adrenal gland itself. In rare instances, ACTH- or cortisol-producing tumors may occur in the body outside the pituitary or adrenal glands themselves.

Manifestations

- The effects of Cushing's syndrome are primarily those of excess cortisol.
- Characteristic "moon face" and "buffalo hump" patterns of fat distribution.
- Glucose intolerance and possible diabetes mellitus.
- Thin skin, poor wound healing, impaired immune function.
- Hypertension.
- Muscle weakness and wasting.
- Reduced bone density, hypercalciuria with possible development of renal calculi.
- Alterations in mental function and personality.
- Increased androgen levels in females with possible "virilization."
- Mortality is approximately 50% within 5 years if left untreated.

Treatment

- Surgical removal of tumors.
- Radiation therapy.
- Chemotherapy if tumor is inoperable. *Mitotane* is a compound that is structurally similar to the insecticide DDT. It is used because of its selective toxicity for cells of the adrenal cortex to treat tumors arising in this tissue.

Disorders of the adrenal medulla

Pheochromocytoma

- A tumor (usually benign) that arises in the *chromaffin* cells of the adrenal medulla that produce the catecholamines.
- Symptoms are those of excess catecholamine production and can be life-threatening.
- Excess catecholamine production may be continual or occur in episodes ("bursts").

Manifestations

- Hypertension
- Tachycardia
- Severe headache
- Nausea and vomiting
- Excess sweating (*diaphoresis*)
- Palpitations
- Anxiety
- Risk of stroke due to marked hypertension

Treatment

- β-Blocking and α-blocking drugs to blunt catecholamine effects
- Surgical removal of tumor

chapter nineteen

Diabetes mellitus

Study objectives

- List the effects of insulin and glucagon in the body.
- List the factors that put an individual at risk for developing diabetes mellitus.
- Discuss the possible etiology of type I and type II diabetes.
- Define the three "polys." Why do they occur?
- What are the manifestations of diabetic ketoacidosis? Why does it occur?
- What is hyperosmolar-hyperglycemic syndrome? Why does it occur?
- Discuss pharmacologic and nonpharmacologic treatment for diabetes mellitus.
- Discuss possible mechanisms of tissue injury in diabetes mellitus.
- List the major effects of chronic diabetes mellitus on the body. Why does each occur?
- Define gestational diabetes.

Introduction

Diabetes mellitus is the most common endocrine disorder. Approximately 800,000 new cases of diabetes are diagnosed each year.[21] The prevalence of diabetes is 8.2% among all men and women in the United States. The frequency of the disease increases to 18.4% in individuals 65 years of age or older. Diabetes is a disease of the *endocrine pancreas*. Some risk factors for diabetes mellitus are presented in Table 19.1.

Table 19.1 Risk Factors for Diabetes Mellitus

Obesity
Familial history of diabetes mellitus
Increasing age
Ethnicity — High risk groups include African–Americans, Hispanics and native Americans
Dietary factors

Endocrine pancreas

Throughout the pancreas there are endocrine cells found in scattered clusters called *islets of Langerhans*. These endocrine cells can be classified into three distinct types: *α cells* that produce the hormone *glucagon*, *β cells* that produce *insulin* and *δ cells* that produce *somatostatin* (see Table 19.2). The major regulator of insulin and glucagon release from the pancreas is the blood glucose level. An increase in blood glucose (as occurs after a meal) will stimulate the release of insulin and inhibit the release of glucagon. Conversely, decreases in blood glucose (during fasting, for example) will stimulate the release of glucagon and inhibit the release of insulin. When released, the main effect of insulin is to lower blood glucose levels by enhancing the utilization and uptake of insulin. Glucagon directly counters the effects of insulin by

Table 19.2 Hormones of the Endocrine Pancreas

Glucagon
Increases glycogen breakdown in liver
Increases lipolysis in adipose tissue
Increases gluconeogenesis in liver
Increases proteolysis in skeletal muscle; liberated amino acids may in turn be converted to glucose
Insulin
Increases glucose transport into tissues
Increases glycogen synthesis in liver and muscle
Increases triglyceride synthesis in adipose tissue and liver
Increases amino acid uptake and protein synthesis
Somatostatin
Inhibits the release of glucagon
Inhibits the release of growth hormone from the anterior pituitary

decreasing glucose utilization and uptake as well as by stimulating the formation of new glucose from glycogen and amino acids. The major target tissues for insulin and glucagon are liver, skeletal muscle and fat.

Types of diabetes mellitus

Type I diabetes (insulin-dependent diabetes)

- Cause appears to be a progressive autoimmune destruction of the pancreatic β cells.
- Most instances of autoimmune pancreatic destruction are idiopathic, but some may occur following viral infections.
- Little or no insulin secretion occurs.

Manifestations

- Hyperglycemia
- Weight loss
- The three "polys" — *polydypsia* (increased thirst), *polyphagia* (increased appetite), *polyuria* (increased urine output)
- Weakness and fatigue due to poor energy utilization and skeletal muscle catabolism
- Diabetic ketoacidosis — Accumulation of acidic ketone bodies in the blood due to a lack of insulin-stimulated fatty acid utilization (see Tables 19.3 and 19.4).
- *Hyperglycemic hyperosmolar syndrome* (see Table 19.5).

Why do the three "polys" occur?

- Polyuria — Excess blood glucose filtered by the kidneys cannot be reabsorbed and is eliminated at the expense of water.
- Polydyspsia — Excessive thirst caused by the osmotic diuresis of glucose and subsequent tissue dehydration. The thirst response is mediated by the hypothalamus.
- Polyphagia — Poor utilization of carbohydrates (due to the lack of insulin) results in depletion of stored fats, proteins and carbohydrates.

Treatment

- Insulin replacement therapy (see Table 19.6)
- Dietary management

Table 19.3 Diabetic Ketoacidosis

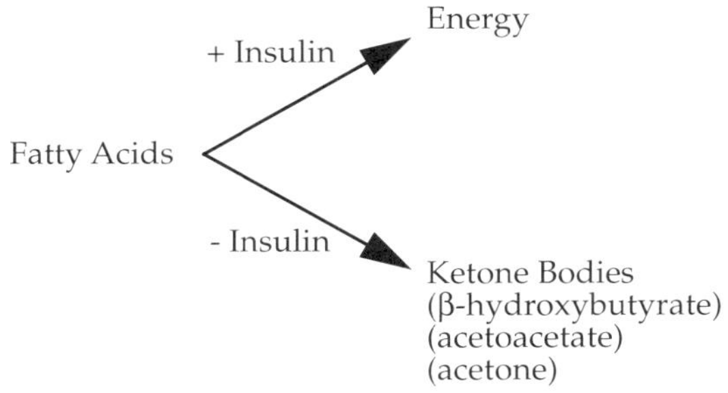

Table 19.4 Manifestations of Diabetic Ketoacidosis

Decreased blood pH levels
Ketonuria — Appearance of excess ketones in the urine
Lethargy
Anorexia
Nausea and vomiting
Markedly increased respiratory rate as an attempt to correct decreased blood pH
Acetone breath — Acetone is a volatile ketone body that is eliminated via the lungs; may be noticeable in the exhaled air during diabetic ketoacidosis
Coma and possible death

Table 19.5 Hyperglycemic Hyperosmolar Syndrome

A syndrome of type I diabetes mellitus that can result from acute insulin deficiency. It may often accompany diabetic ketoacidosis. The manifestations include:
Severe dehydration
Extreme thirst
Serum osmolarity over 300 mOsm due to excessive glucose in the blood
Osmotic diuresis of glucose
Depressed neurologic function
Possible shock, coma and death

Table 19.6 Insulin Therapy

Insulin preparations were originally derived from bovine or porcine sources but now are supplied as a pure human form made by recombinant DNA technology or modification of porcine insulin. Insulin must be administered by injection because an oral form would be degraded in the gastrointestinal tract. Insulin is generally available in three preparations:
Short-acting form — Peak action in 2–4 hours, duration 6–8 hours.
Intermediate-acting form — Peak action in 6–12 hours, duration 12–24 hours.
Long-acting form — Peak action 8–24 hours, duration 24–36 hours.

Type II diabetes mellitus (non-insulin-dependent diabetes)

- Greater prevalence than type I diabetes.
- The primary manifestation is "insulin resistance," which is a lack of responsiveness by tissues and the pancreas itself to insulin. The exact etiology of the insulin resistance is unknown but may be linked to abnormalities of insulin receptors, intracelluar signaling pathways or glucose transporters.
- Insulin resistance may be related to increased levels of free fatty acids (FFA) that stimulate insulin secretions and inhibit glucose uptake by tissues (Figure 19.1). FFAs are elevated in obese individuals with a predisposition to type II diabetes.

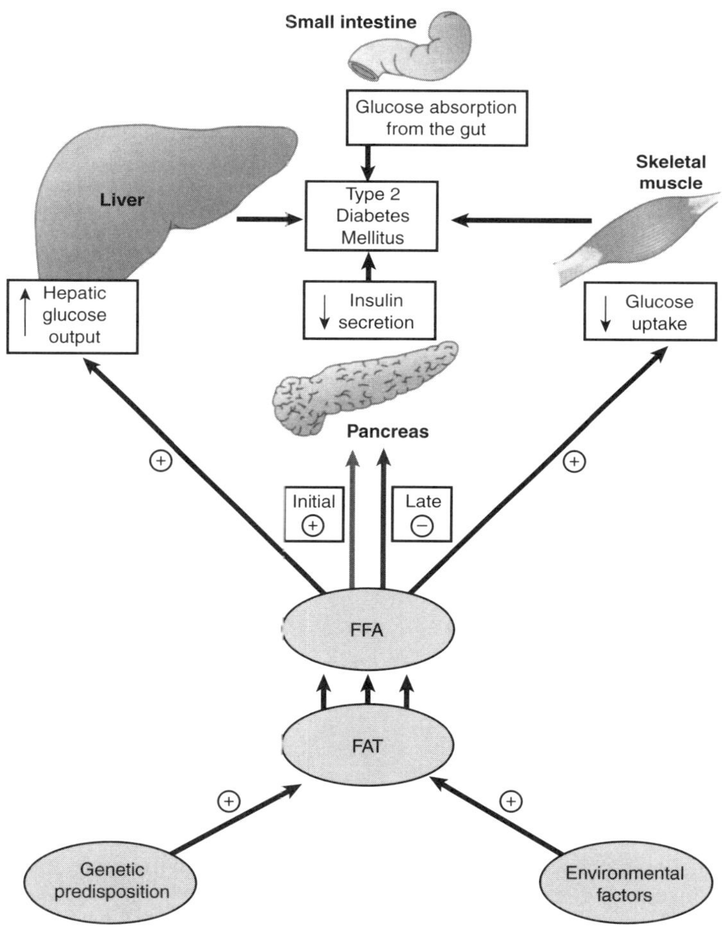

Figure 19.1 Pathogenesis of type II diabetes. FFA = free fatty acids. (From Porth, C.M., *Pathophysiology: Concepts of Altered Health States*, 5th ed., Lippincott, Philadelphia, 1998. With permission.)

- Obesity appears to be an important contributing factor to development of type II diabetes.[22] Tissues (liver, fat and muscle) in obese individuals have an altered responsiveness to the effects of insulin.
- A strong genetic component is also present.[23]
- Insulin secretion may be normal or even elevated at the time of diagnosis.
- The continued overproduction of insulin by the β cells can eventually lead to β-cell "burnout" and destruction.

Manifestations

Manifestations of type II diabetes may include many of those seen in type I diabetes including polyuria, polydypsia, polyphagia, fatigue and weakness. Other manifestations of type II diabetes tend to be more generalized:

- Hyperinsulinemia
- Visual changes
- *Parasthesias* (abnormal sensations such as tingling or burning, often occur in the extremities)
- Recurrent infections
- Ketoacidosis is rare with type II diabetes

Treatment

- Weight loss has been reported to improve insulin sensitivity in obese individuals with type II diabetes.[24]
- Exercise may enhance glucose utilization and improve glucose control in patients with type II diabetes, thus reducing the risk of diabetic complications.[25]
- Dietary management.
- Oral hypoglycemic drugs (see Table 19.7).
- Insulin-replacement may be necessary during later stages of the disease when β cells are destroyed in order to maintain normal metabolic function (see Table 19.6).

Table 19.7 Oral Hypoglycemic Drugs

Sulfonylureas (example: glipizide)
Simulate insulin secretion from the β cells
Only effective if some β cells are still functional
Biguanides (example: metformin)
Act peripherally to increase glucose uptake by skeletal muscle, provided some insulin is still present
Thiazolidinedione derivatives (example: pioglitazone)
Increase insulin sensitivity in peripheral tissues
Increase glucose uptake and oxidation in muscle and adipose tissues independent of insulin

Long-term complications of diabetes mellitus

There are a number of long-term complications of diabetes mellitus that contribute significantly to the mortality and morbidity that is seen with this disease. The etiology of the complications is likely multifactorial and involves tissue injury related to chronically elevated blood glucose levels. Some possible causes of tissue injury in chronic diabetes mellitus are listed in Table 19.8. The occurrence of these long-term complications can be greatly reduced by proper management of blood glucose levels.

Chronic diabetes mellitus can lead to injury in a number of different target organs including the kidney, eye, blood vessels and nervous system.

1. Diabetic neuropathy
   - Most common cause of neuropathy in the United States.
   - Abnormality of nerve conduction and function.
   - Often affects peripheral nerves.
   - Can involve sensory or motor neurons.
   - May manifest as numbness, pain or sensory/motor impairment.
   - Often progressive and irreversible.
   - Although the exact cause is unknown, the neuropathy may be related to ischemia or altered nerve cell metabolism.
2. Diabetic nephropathy
   - Diabetes is the leading cause of end-stage renal disease in the United States.
   - Glomerular injury is the key feature of diabetic nephropathy. The glomerular injury is characterized by thickening of the glomerular basement membrane and *glomerulosclerosis*.
   - Although the exact etiology is unclear, trapping of glycosylated proteins in the glomeruli appears to be a key contributing factor.
   - The appearance of protein (albumin) in the urine is an early indicator of altered glomerular permeability.

Table 19.8 Possible Mechanisms of Tissue Injury in Chronic Diabetes Mellitus

Glycosylation of proteins — Attachment of glucose to proteins in the eye, blood vessel walls, and kidney membranes will change their structure and may lead to altered function and eventual damage of these tissues. Circulating glycosylated proteins may also be trapped in the glomeruli of the kidney, leading to inflammation and injury.
Formation of alcohol sugars (example: sorbitol) — Unlike glucose, alcohol sugars do not easily diffuse out of tissues. Because these alcohol sugars are osmotically active, they can lead to swelling and damage of tissues. The accumulation of other sugars such as galactose might also contribute to this phenomenon.
Poor blood flow and oxygen delivery to tissues — Glycosylation of hemoglobin alters its affinity for oxygen while progressive vascular disease can reduce overall blood flow to tissues, leading to ischemic injury.

Table 19.9 Diagnosis and Monitoring of Diabetes Mellitus

Diagnosis of diabetes
Often evident due to the three "polys," as well as significant weight loss
Elevated fasting blood glucose levels (>140 mg/dL)
Presence of glucose in the urine
Monitoring of diabetes
Frequent measurement of blood glucose levels
Measurement of *glycosylated hemoglobin* (Hb A_{1c}, hemoglobin that has glucose bound to it) that forms at a rate that increases with increasing blood glucose, which is a useful measure of blood glucose control in patients with diabetes
Measurement of urine ketone levels in patients with insulin-dependent diabetes mellitus is also useful to assess disease management

- Renal function may continue to deteriorate as glomerular filtration decreases. Signs and symptoms of renal insufficiency will appear as renal function continues to decline.

3. Vascular disease
   - Chronic diabetes mellitus is associated with significant increases in the incidence of coronary artery disease, cerebrovascular disease and peripheral vascular disease.
   - May be due to a number of factors including elevated serum lipid levels, vascular injury, and enhanced atherogenesis (formation of atherosclerotic lesions).
   - Coronary artery disease and stroke are significant sources of mortality and morbidity in patients with diabetes. Peripheral vascular disease can lead to gangrene and amputations (particularly of the toes and feet) in people suffering from diabetes.
4. Impaired healing and increased infections risk
   - As a result of peripheral vascular disease, injuries in patients with diabetes do not heal properly. Poor blood flow limits the delivery of leukocytes and oxygen to the injured area while impairing removal of debris and infectious organisms.
   - The high glucose levels serve as a nutrient to support the growth of microorganisms.
   - Patients with diabetes might also be more susceptible to physical injuries as a result of impaired vision and sensory perception.
5. Diabetic retinopathy
   - Diabetes mellitus is the leading cause of acquired blindness in the United States.
   - The most serious consequence of long-term diabetes in terms of the eye is retinal damage. The retina is a highly metabolic tissue that is especially vulnerable to the effects of chronic hypoxia and diabetes. Hemorrhage of eye capillaries and chronic inflammation is common and can lead to increases in intraocular pressure that scar the retina and impair vision. This phenomenon is usually progressive and can lead to blindness.

- Diabetes is also associated with an increased incidence of glaucoma and cataract formation.

Gestational diabetes

- Glucose intolerance in about 1 to 6% of pregnancies.
- May present with variable severity.
- Most commonly seen during the third trimester of pregnancy.
- Resolves itself in most patients after birth but a certain percentage (50 to 60%) will go on to develop diabetes mellitus in the years following the pregnancy.
- May be associated with an increased risk of fetal abnormalities.
- Currently recommended that all pregnant women be screened for the presence of gestational diabetes.

References

1. Sharma, S. and Dastroy, S.K. Images in clinical medicine. Gingival hyperplasia induced by phenytoin. *New England Journal of Medicine*, 342:325, 2000.
2. Butterfield, D.A., Drake, J., Poernich, C., et al. Evidence of oxidative damage in Alzeheimer's diseased brain: central role for amyloid beta-peptide. *Trends in Molecular Medicine*, 7:548–554, 2001.
3. Spiteller, G. Lipid peroxidation in aging and age-dependent diseases. *Experimental Gerontology*. 36:1425–1457, 2001.
4. American Cancer Society 2001 Surveillance Report, available at www.cancer.org.
5. Shen, Y. and White, E., p53-Dependent apoptosis pathways. *Advances in Cancer Research*, 82:55–84, 2001.
6. Peters, J., Loud, J., Dimond, E., et al. Cancer genetics fundamentals. *Cancer Nursing*, 24:446–461, 2001.
7. Keller, U. Pathophysiology of cancer cachexia. *Support Care in Cancer*, 1:290–294, 1993.
8. Lucarelli, G., Andreani, M., and Angeluccie, E. The cure of thalassemia with bone marrow transplantation. *Bone Marrow Transplantation*, 28(Suppl. 1):S11–13, 2001.
9. Centers for Disease Control at www.cdc.gov, 2002.
10. Mellors, J.W., Munoz, A., Giorgi, J.V., et al. Plasma viral load and CD4+ lymphocytes as prognostic markers of HIV-1 infection. *Annals of Internal Medicine*, 126:946–954, 1997.
11. Durant, J., Clevebergh, P., Halfon, P., et al. Drug-resistance genotyping in HIV-1 drug therapy: The VIRADAPT randomized controlled trial. *Lancet*, 353:2195–2199, 1999.
12. American Heart Association, at *americanheart.org/presenter*, 2002.
13. Hunt, H.A., et al. ACC/AHA Guidelines for the evaluation and management of chronic heart failure in the adult. *Circulation*, 104:2996–3019, 2001.
14. Guyton, A.C. and Hall, J.E. Heart muscle; the heart as a pump, in *Human Physiology and Mechanisms of Disease*, 6th ed., W.B. Saunders, Philadelphia, 1997, p. 91.
15. Cohn, J.N., The management of chronic heart failure. *New England Journal of Medicine*. 325:490–498, 1996.
16. Levy, S.B. The challenge of antibiotic resistance. *Scientific American*, Mar:46–53, 1998.

17. Bartlett, J.G., et al. Community-acquired pneumonia in adults: guidelines for management. *Clinical Infectious Disease*, 26:811–838, 1998.
18. Pulmonary disorders, in *The Merck Manual*, 16th ed., R. Berkow, Ed., Merck Research Laboratories, Rahway, NJ, 1992, p. 648.
19. Main, J. and Thomas, H. Interferons in chronic viral hepatitis, in *Clinical Applications of the Interferons*, R. Stuart-Harris and R.D. Penny, Eds., Chapman & Hall, London, 1997, pp. 53–66.
20. Zdanowicz, M. Human growth hormone: ethical and economical considerations of use and misuse. *Journal of Managed Care Pharmacy*, 3:448–452, 1997.
21. National Diabetes Information Clearinghouse, at www.niddk.nih, 2002.
22. Zimmet, P., Alberti, K.G., and Shaw, J. Global and societal implications of the diabetes epidemic. *Nature*, 414:782–787, 2001.
23. Gloyn, A.L. and McCarthy, M.I. The genetics of type 2 diabetes. *Best Practice & Research Clinical Endocrinology & Metabolism*, 15:293–308, 2001.
24. Boule, N.G., Haddad, E., Kenny, G.P., et al. Effects of exercise on glycemic control and body mass in type 2 diabetes mellitus: a meta-analysis of controlled clinical trials. *Journal of the American Medical Association*, 286:1218–1227, 2001.
25. Bonora, E. Relationship between regional fat distribution and insulin resistance. *International Journal of Obesity*, 24(Suppl. 2):S32–35, 2000.

Selected bibliography

Boyd, R.F. *Basic Medical Microbiology,* 5th ed., Little, Brown, Boston, 1995.

Brook, C.G.D. and Marshall, N.J. *Essential Endocrinology,* 4th ed., Blackwell Sciences, Oxford, U.K., 2001.

Hardman, J.E., Limbird, L.E., and Gilman, A.G., Eds., Goodman and Gilman's *Pharmacological Basis of Therapeutics,* 10th ed., McGraw-Hill, New York, 2001.

Katzung, B.G., Ed., *Basic & Clinical Pharmacology,* 8th ed., Lange, New York, 2001.

McCance, K. and Huether, S.E. *Pathophysiology: The Biologic Basis for Disease in Adults and Children,* 3rd ed., Mosby, St. Louis, MO, 1998.

Porth, C.M. Heart failure and circulatory shock, in *Pathophysiology: Concepts of Altered Health States,* 5th ed., Lippincott, Philadelphia, 1998, pp. 427–456.

Price, S.A. and Wilson, L.M. *Pathophysiology: Clinical Concepts of Disease Processes,* 5th ed., Mosby, St. Louis, MO, 1997.

Index

A

B

D

E

F

G

H

I

N

O

V

W

X

Z